It's Positively Cancer

I0091265

It's Positively Cancer

a daughter's blog, a dad's farewell

Andy Smith

Tracy Lynn Hamilton

TKR Publishing
Nashville, TN

copyright@2017 TKR Publishing #1-6055465041 Nashville, Tennessee

Contents

It's Positively Cancer

A DAUGHTER'S BLOG

A DAD'S FAREWELL

by Andy Smith

Dedication

To the employees and regulars at
The Village Pub & Beer Garden
in East Nashville, TN who made it possible for
Jesse, Tracy and the family
to support Tracy throughout this ordeal.
You cried with us
laughed with us
you kept the Pub going.
Your support is greatly appreciated...
THANK YOU

Introduction

a daughter's blog, a dad's farewell

ANDY SMITH

My daughter, Tracy Hamilton, started a facebook blog page when she found out she had Stage III breast cancer. She wanted it to be a platform for her to write about her journey and to possibly connect with others along the way. Her and her husband, Jesse, owned a popular bar in East Nashville, and she didn't want to have to answer questions about her health all the time and felt this blog would be a good source for her regulars, family and friends to keep up with her journey.

When her journey was over, it was always my desire to put her blog into a book form so that anyone who wanted could get a copy of her story. And her story is in the attitude and character she displayed as a young mother, wife and business woman as she took on the challenge of her life …. and eventually, her death.

People needed to hear her story, and though it was three years after her passing before I could emotionally deal with it, once I committed to it, the story pretty much wrote itself.

I'm happy – and sad – to share this story with others. Those who read it will understand why I have always considered myself the richest man in the world.

1

My Daughter My Best Friend

I have said it many times, and will continue to do so until I pass, that if you want to create a designer family you would need to start with Tracy as your oldest child.

Tracy did not have a bad stage in her thirty-seven years on this planet. That's not to say she was an angel – quite the contrary. She could go toe to toe with her father, and being her Dad, I can honestly say there were many times I would be frustrated while debating her and thinking, "Why can't you just say 'Okay Dad, and move on? Why do you have to make such a good argument!?"

To my credit, I did fairly well for a guy who hates to argue. There were more than a few occasions when I would remind her that even tough the rule we debated may not be applicable to her, it was important to remember that there are a couple of ears down the hall listening to see if big sister can win the battle and save their hides from future battles.

As a parent it seemed to me that it was an important code of conduct in being a good parent that you are consistent with the rules. One rule fits all. Even though, as the 5th child in a family of 6, I well remember that by the time I became a teenager, the only rule I ever got was, 'Just don't kill yourself, alright!' I do believe that my older brothers still have a hint of resentment towards me because as a teenager during the wild '60s, I sure had a lot of fun with very few consequences.

That's what makes being the oldest child such a pain. I got that 'look' from Tracy more times than I care to remember that screamed at me, "OH, I SEE HOW IT IS .... " well, you can fill in the blanks here as I still get too emotional just thinking about it. But to my credit, as the great Dad that I was, I quickly responded to that look with, "Awwww, does Tracy need a hug? Come to papa", which was greeted by another look that I frankly have no desire to share with anyone. That girl had a look that could back off a hungry bear.

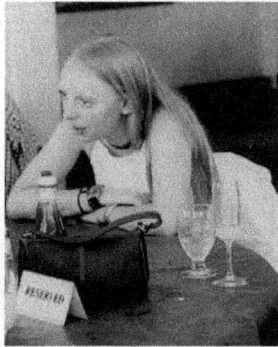

She could give you that look,
trust me

You'd think that parents would get this right by now. This very minute there are two people putting down this book because they can't read through their tears of laughter – all parents, and all siblings who were not the oldest child. Those of you who are still with me are the oldest child in a multi-level family who are now rolling your eyes and screaming at me, "THAT'S NO JOKE, BUB!"

You see, generation after generation, parents have lived under this code of being consistent, which is a good thing. The problem is that they almost always choose the very worst things to be consistent with. Common sense will tell everyone who is not a parent that consistency has no place in rules. Common sense tells us you don't make a rule unless you have a problem. If you don't have a problem, you don't need a rule. And you never, ever establish a rule assuming that there may be a problem somewhere down the road a couple of kids from now.

When I talk about being a consistent parent, it has nothing to do with the mechanics of life. The rules, tasks and schedules that give us gray hair will never be consistent – and should NEVER be. You are always adjusting if you are a good parent to every moment and making decisions based on that moment and what is in the best interest of your child. Being locked into a consistent, non-negotiated set of rules for all children regardless of need will never be in the best interest of a child at any particular moment of time.

What makes a good parent is being consistent on an emotional level. That does not mean always perky or always grumpy, it means that the more predictable you are in their eyes, the more relaxed they are in meeting the challenges of growing up in this world.

I'll give you an example.

As a struggling single parent, it was not a stretch for me to sometimes let the girls eat their dinner in the living room while watching the Muppet show or a Bugs Bunny special(trust me – it was my idea as I loved watching those shows). It was not a stretch to find us eating dinner in the dinning room and catching up with all that was going on in their worlds. It was also not a stretch to find me grabbing some PB&J sandwiches and fruit and heading for an evening at the beach.

Now there are a lot of people with a string of important letters by their name that would suggest that I was very inconsistent in my parenting skills which was unhealthy for my girls.

Of course, I would suggest that they are full of baloney.

My daughters grew up to be very healthy young ladies because they absolutely knew who their Dad was and how he would respond to any given situation. It wasn't that I was an emotional Dad, but that I was honest with my emotions. My daughters may not know from day to day where they would eat their dinner, but they always knew their Dad was emotionally honest and they could be comfortable with him no matter what.

I suppose that's why Tracy was so willing to go toe to toe with me when she started crashing in on her teen years. She knew her Dad hated conflict and if she stood her ground and made a good argument, she had a fair chance of reversing the ruling – which I did on many occasions without apologies.

That's the problem with parenting. I did pretty good when the girls were cute little darlings, but when Tracy hit 13, it's like this gene inside of me exploded and wiped out all my common sense and drove me to become a complete lunatic holding on to rules that will save my precious child from the horrors of being a teenager. The horrors of being a teenager has nothing to do with the kids and everything to do with the parents having exploding genes that go off when your child blows out those 13 candles.

Like I said earlier, I was a teenager in the '60s and though I certainly had a lot of fun going to all the concerts, the beaches and generally living the good life as a San Diego teenager, I didn't get into any trouble. Tried some drugs, but was never impressed and stopped before I started, really. Didn't take advantage of women or tried to hurt anyone – was actually a pretty shy guy when it came to the ladies. I was just a happy guy living the fun life that came wrapped up in '60s clothing. A hippie. A surfer. A womanizer wannabe. A protester.

But my parents always taught me to be considerate. Care about others. Not to be selfish. I guess it was in being the 5th child. By the time they got to me, that gene had already exploded and washed out of their system, I suppose.

Tracy really was a good kid. I enjoyed being her Dad more and more with every year I was given with her. By the time she got cancer, she truly was my best friend as much – if not more so – than my daughter.

I am not embellishing my words when I say that Tracy had every good reason to become a rebellious, obnoxious teenager, given the hand that she was dealt. Her biological mother left us when she was very young. I kid you not when I tell you that the Judge in the divorce hearing told me – and I can pretty much be exact here – "Mr Smith, I have no reason to believe that you will be successful. Their mother makes more than you and has a stable job, they are girls and there is no prospects in your future to give me hope that the girls will be well provided for. But since there is no one here to challenge you, I have no choice but to wish you luck and give you custody of these girls." Not a ringing endorsement of confidence, I know, but I got the girls, and in the late 1970s, a man who was a dreamer with little business talent and even less financial prospects, getting custody of the girls was all I was looking for.

To be honest, I couldn't argue one point of what the judge had told me. He was absolutely right. But when the marriage started to melt down, I made it very clear that my wife was welcome to leave and take whatever she wanted from our home, but I got the kids. I would not negotiate that.

Now even though it was California in the late '70s, being a single parent Dad was pretty unheard of. Poor Tracy was stuck with a Dad who was the poster boy for starving writers who had no guarantees of making it as a songwriter, but was always willing to take them to the beach to get away from the bill collector calls. I was a parent like I was a baseball player in my youth. I played with 80% heart and 20% skills. Tracy had to adjust many times to her loveable Dad trying hard to make it all work for us as a family. To say she had a normal upbringing is a ridicules thing to say. There was nothing normal about our lives.

I had a publisher I was working with in L.A. tell me that I'd probably do better if I lived in Nashville, TN. So after watching some episodes of Hee Haw, I announced to the girls that when Tracy finished 1st grade, we would be moving to Nashville, TN where I have never been, had no prospects for jobs and had no clue what a dry county was, how grits tasted, or that Nashville was the buckle of the Bible belt.

In 1983, I packed up my 1969 square back VW station wagon (which- I'm not making this up – had no dials on the dashboard that worked) full of barbie dolls, toys, blankets, pillows and my guitar and headed through the deserts, hills and valleys with no air conditioning in late June, to be discovered in Music City USA.

It made sense to me.

I brush off others who ask me now how I did it back then, because I seriously have no idea how we survived. But I do know that I couldn't have done any of it without Tracy. So willing to roll with the flow of a crazy Dad pursuing his dreams. There were no tantrums when there probably should have been. There were no whiny fits when she would have likely been justified. She was never moody or quick to anger. And her little sister, Kelly, worshiped her big sister and even at that young age, Tracy had a pretty good sense of understanding that it would be best if she helped Kelly out with any of the issues of the day as her Dad was too busy trying to figure out why phone calls were still coming from bill collectors and not country music stars looking for a great song.

She was the best oldest child a Dad could ask for without question. She saved my butt and I don't mean that lightly. I often thought of how I would have handled the same circumstances in my youth and there is no question in my mind that I would have been horrible. I truly admired my daughter long before she even became a teenager.

She was special when I desperately needed someone special to help me get through all the rough spots.

I remember when Tracy was in 2nd grade – her first year in Nashville – I went to a parent/teacher meeting with Mrs Davis. She was going through all the subjects they were studying and mentioned that maybe her mother could work with Tracy on some math scales they were going to be doing, when I interrupted her and informed her that she didn't have a mother, that it was just me, Tracy and Kelly. Mrs Davis sat back in her chair and looked at me for what certainly seemed like an uncomfortable amount of time before saying, "Mr Smith, had anyone else told me that Tracy came from a single parent setting, I would never have believed it"

That was Tracy.

Then there was the time I took the girls to the San Diego

Zoo shortly before we moved. Kelly had to go to the bathroom and being fairly new to the diaper-free society, it put me in an awkward position. They were both a tad too old to be going into the mens room with me, but I wasn't real keen about sending them into the ladies room alone. So I instructed Tracy to go with her sister and stay together, do not talk to anyone, do your business, wash your hands and come out to me without saying anything to anyone.

While I was waiting nervously outside, these two old ladies came out and stood next to me, talking about the two girls in the bathroom all alone.

" Do you mean the blonde and the redhead in there?"

"Why yes"

"Did they misbehave towards you?"

"Well no, but those girls are way too young to be in there without their mother!"

I looked her straight in the eyes and said, "I am their mother … do I need to go in there?"

The ladies flustered away without further conversation.

When the girls came out, I asked Tracy if they had any problems. Tracy, with her thumb ever present in her mouth, pulled the plug and announced, " Some lady kept asking me questions." Thumb back in mouth.

"What did you say to her?"

Tracy looked at me (yes, she had 'that look' even then), shrugged her shoulders, removed her plug and said, mater of factly, " Nothing – you told me not to talk to anyone."

I laughed so hard I was almost in tears as I took them over to get an ice cream for being such good sports.

That was Tracy.

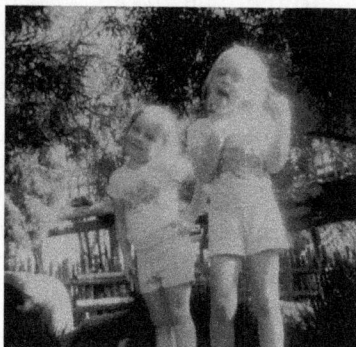

Tracy & Kelly having fun at San Diego Zoo

As an old, retired man today, I often look back on the journey I have had and still have no idea how I made it all work out. I still think that what the Judge told me so many years ago was true. I never had a desire to prove the Judge wrong because I never thought he was. I was just too busy trying to survive in a crazy world of being a dreamer, a single Dad and man with a heart of Peter Pan who never wanted to grow up in the first place.

But I had Tracy on my side and that is the only explanation I can come to. She kept me going. She gave me the confidence that as long as she was on my side, I could be a winner in this world of parenting. As long as I had Tracy that my other daughters could look up to and follow, I knew I would be okay.

She was my rock. She was my T-Rock long before her friends ordained her as T-Rock when she was an adult. And she was called T-Rock by them for the very same reasons she was my T-Rock, and that says about all you need to know about my daughter.

2

Introduction - Tracy

My name is Tracy Hamilton and I was diagnosed with Stage III breast cancer in January 2012. After a biopsy and test results telling me what kind I have, PET and CAT scans, and a port-a-cath put in, I began chemo treatments 2 1/2 weeks later starting with Adriamycin and Cytoxan every 2 weeks for 8 weeks then Taxol every week for 12 weeks. After that, on July 31, 2012 I had a double mastectomy (even though the tumor was found only in the right breast) and then 6 weeks of radiation that fall to make sure it is all gone.

My doctors and nurses have been telling me that a positive attitude works healing wonders when dealing with cancer. So while they are treating me with drugs and surgery, I'll be doing my part by finding the laughter and positive outlook when facing each challenge presented to me.

Even though I have started this page to give myself an outlet through this journey, I also want to bring awareness to breast cancer in younger women. My doctors have told me that this is a "55 year old woman's disease", even though it is not completely uncommon in younger women. Most gynecologist don't give their patients a mammogram until they are 40 years old. I caught mine because I was breast-feeding, but I did not catch it in an early stage. I want to encourage all women to do regular breast exams on themselves and if you are unsure about ANYTHING, check it out with your doctor. It could mean everything.

3

The Journey Begins

It's Positively Cancer

February 12, 2012

Hello to the Facebook world! This is the beginning of my journey through the LONG process of fighting (and beating!) breast cancer. Facebookers beware – it's not gonna be pretty, but in the end I WILL prevail! Thank you for coming along.

(and no, that is not my tattoo – at least, not yet.)

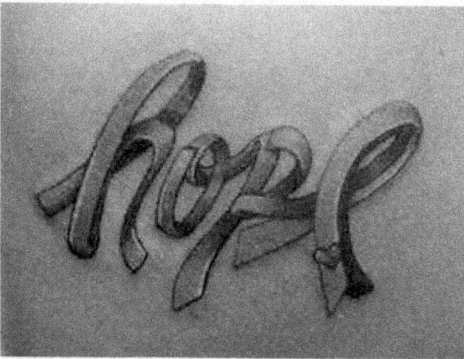

It's Positively Cancer
February 13, 2012
Shortly after my first chemo treatment (which was 2 weeks and 3 days ago), in anticipation of losing my hair, I went to my favorite hair stylist and cut my long hair that I have had for years to just below my chin. This is pretty short for me, but I figured, why not, right? Try something new! What do I have to lose?

It's Positively Cancer
February 14, 2012
2nd chemo treatment on Valentine's Day – what?! Not the most romantic setting for our afternoon away from the baby, but you make the best of it – with lunch at the Goldrush and buying books afterward!
Not sure how romantic the Goldrush is either, though……..hmmmm. Still, it's lunch! I gotta take advantage while food still tastes good, right?! Happy Valentine's Day to me!

It's Positively Cancer
February 15, 2012
Doc told me yesterday that it feels like the tumor has shrunk some (even after 1 chemo treatment!!) and that it probably looks like Swiss cheese instead of one big mass. YAY – take THAT tumor!
I personally like to envision chemo as an army of small

soldiers shooting rifles at the tumor making the holes in it....I mean, it IS a war we are fighting (plus I think I saw a mouthwash or a flea treatment commercial with these guys fightin' bad breath or ticks recently, so it's on the brain. Advertising DOES work!)

Anyway, good news!

It's Positively Cancer
February 16, 2012

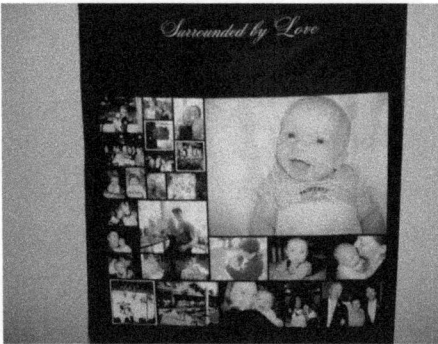

A Blanket of LOVE

This is a blanket my friend Lauren made for me to take to chemo and just have around to lift my spirits!

It's Positively Cancer
February 18, 2012

It's crazy that a stressful day would normally put me in a cranky mood and make me want to run home and eat something that doesn't match like leftover spaghetti and tater tots, junk out to some God-awful TV show that I would never watch EVER (I'm talking to YOU, America's Next Top Model Marathon!), and drink a 6-pack of high-alcohol Sweetwater IPA just to cleanse myself of the day.

But now, this stressful day has given me a gift – I was so busy, I forgot all day long that I have cancer! SWEET! I'll take this kind of stress any day!.........aaannnd maybe that 6-pack too!

It's Positively Cancer
February 17, 2012

So I'm trying my best to hold on to the hair until Sunday night. I've got a baby shower to go to Sunday afternoon and I just don't want to roll up with a cleanly shaved head and shock the hell out of my friend and put her into labor early. But I'm not sure if showing up all patchy is the right way to go either. I'd feel like some doll that that mean kid from "Toy Story 1" made that freaked out Woody and the gang (even though they were REALLY nice when you got to know them!). It's a tough call..........

It's Positively Cancer
February 20, 2012

A question for my fellow bald friends or friends of bald friends from the newly shaven (that's me!) – How do you tidy up the look? I'm trying to go for the Mr. Clean sleek-and-shiny, but having some trouble taking it all off. Wax it (!)?....ouch! Plus, how do you take care of a bald head? Moisturize? Is there a head tonic or something I don't know about? I'm so new at this – ANYTHING is helpful!!!

It's Positively Cancer
February 21, 2012
The Hair Evolution!

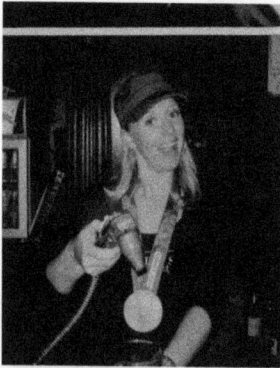

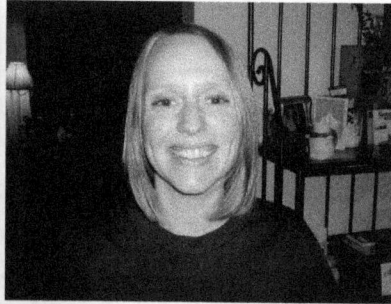

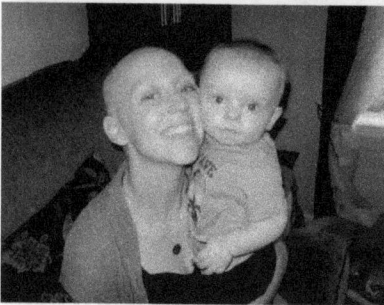

It's Positively Cancer
February 23, 2012
The past few days have been rough. There has been a lot of stress and sleepless nights (mostly un-cancer related) and my

morale has taken a bit of a blow. So what do you do when life gets you down? (Ladies, you know what I'm about to say.......)

YOU GO SHOPPING!

Now, I'm not a shopping kinda girl. I'm more of a get-in, buy, and get-out type of person and it's usually for the basics or the necessaries and most of the time not for me. But, I figured my new 'do needed a wardrobe update, so momma spent some money on herself! And I must admit, it was quite therapeutic! Shopping, you and I may become friends after all.

It's Positively Cancer
February 25, 2012

To the anonymous sender of the package I have received this week, I want to say thank you. I am truly at a loss for words. You are too generous and kind and you make me want to be a more thoughtful, giving person. I wish I could send you cookies at the very least or give you a BIG HUG to express my gratitude. Thank you again from the bottom of my heart. Tracy

It's Positively Cancer
February 27, 2012

I figured that I would have a bit of a struggle getting used to how I look with no hair since I have never been bald before. Sometimes I feel self-conscious, but mostly I just feel a bit surprised when I catch my reflection in the mirror or see it in a window. It seems that while other people who see me often are getting used to it, it still jumps out to me as being a bit shocking.

So last night Jesse and I were watching the Oscars (I'm an awards show junkie!!)and looking at all the beautiful starlets dressed in ball gowns and looking better than normal. I'm sure that every woman feels slightly frumpy compared to these gorgeous women at times, but I really started to be conscious of my bald head and my drool-stained shirt. THEN, Angelina Jolie gets on stage in a slinky black number with a sexy slit up to her thigh, a gorgeous bright red smile on those pouty lips of hers, and a beaming Brad Pitt staring up at her. Just as I was about to sink into the couch, grab a hat to hide the head, and start thinking how weird I look, Jesse says from the other end of the couch (unprovoked):

"I don't understand what all the hype is about. She is too skinny – look at her arms."

Best. Husband. Ever.

It's Positively Cancer
February 28, 2012

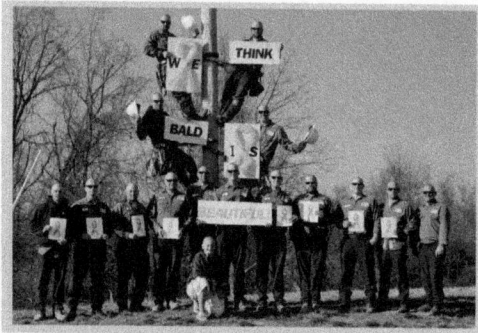

How AWESOME is this picture! These men live in Arkansas and only Matt – the tall guy in the middle, who is my cousin Lea Ann's husband – knows me. Some of them were already rockin' the shaved head look, but the others had a shaving party and took this picture for me. How AMAZING are people – I'm not a crier, but I look at this and tear up. Thanks for the support you guys! I LOVE IT!

It's Positively Cancer
March 1, 2012

Third regiment of chemo under my belt! 3 down and 13 to go ……. yuck!

As I try to remain positive, I am trying to take pleasure out of the little things in life (as one is want to do in situations like this). I started listing things in my head of what really makes me happy or brings me joy. Aside from the obvious – Charlie, Jesse, my family and friends – here is the list I got started:

Friday at the mailbox when I get my issue of Entertainment Weekly!

Hockey!

Taco night!

A glass of really hoppy beer (preferably a Pale Ale or IPA)…..make that a TALL glass!

The Delilah Show on Mix 92.9 after 7pm – she is the self-proclaimed Queen of Sappy Love songs and makes me laugh with her corny, wholesome banter!

"Finding Nemo"!

The Harry Potter books (and yes, I know I'm 35 years old and they are kids books, but I love them anyway!)

Making Charlie laugh ……. I had to throw ONE Charlie-brings-me-joy example!

Kisses from Jesse……I couldn't help that one either!

PIZZA!!!

PIZZA and BEER!!!!

Still have the list taking shape, but this is a good start!

It's Positively Cancer
March 9, 2012

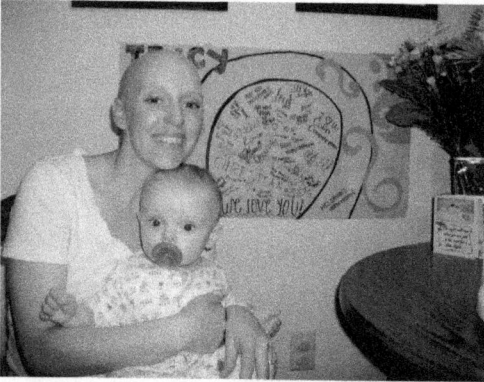

My mom's home room class made me this poster wishing me well, so I hung it up in my kitchen to see every day! How awesome are kids – thanks you guys!

It's Positively Cancer
March 15, 2012

Chemo Treatment #4, done and DONE! This was the last of the heavy duty drugs with the worst side effects, whew! The next round is 12 weeks of Taxol (I think I spelled that right), which is easier for your system to handle, even though it will be given to me every week instead of every other week. Apparently, the main side effect with this round is a feeling of being drunk, which sounds a heck of a lot better than being nauseous!!

Now, according to my calculations, the last chemo treatmeant I will have (barring any set-back of any kind) will be June 19th.....which is something of a problem for me. I have been told that surgery will follow that, which is fine and expected. However, I am getting a bit concerned with the timing of it all, merely because it may fall right SMACK into the Stanley Cup FINALS and there is NO WAY I am going to miss the Preds vying for the Cup! I know, I know........I'm a big hockey nerd to even be thinking about that right now. But my doctors have been stressing the importance of living a normal life through this and I'll be damned if cancer will get in the way of witnessing my beloved Predators as Stanley Cup Champs! I don't want to look back on this experience and have to think, "wellp, sure I beat cancer, but I missed the Preds in the FINAL ROUND because I was laid up in bed watching on TV while everyone else was there in gold, cheering them on". No thanks – I plan on temporarily tattooing my bald head with the Preds logo, dressing Charlie out in his Preds finest, and waving my gold towel in the air IN PERSON!

I might have to have a serious talk with doc.......I'll give cancer the month of July if I can just have June for hockey!!!!! Lucky for me, she is a Preds fan too!

It's Positively Cancer
March 24, 2012

A couple of nights ago, I went to dinner with 3 friends from high school that I don't get a chance to see very often. We had reconnected through the magic of Facebook and this page and decided that too much time had passed since we had seen each other. Luckily we picked a slower night for the restaurant because we ended up being THAT table of girls – we were so engrossed in catching up that it took forever to order drinks, much less food, we took pictures, and totally camped at the table for over 3 hours. (And yes, I felt guilty enough as a restaurant industry vet that I left our sweet server a big tip for taking over her table for so long!) I had a great time and we promised to meet again in a few weeks, opening up the possibility to have even more friends join us (any takers?).

When I get home, Charlie is asleep and Jesse wasn't too far behind, so I decide to take control of the TV and keep my girl-themed night going by grabbing a beer from the fridge, getting into my comfortable (but cute!) summer nightgown, and popping in a DVD of "Sex and the City". Now, when I was in my twenties, this was MY SHOW. My friend Kate introduced me to it and we would have marathon viewings and drink way too much wine while dressing up in feather boas and trying to decide which character we were most like (I was a Carrie-Charlotte hybrid at the time). I eventually bought the whole series on DVD and when I got my own apartment, I would more often than not have it playing on my TV. I could always find an episode that could fit a question or situation that as happening in my life at the time. But, as time went on and I started living with a man, I didn't watch it nearly as much, just settling on an episode here or there that I happened across on the E! network late at night (which are VERY clean versions – I'm talking no F-bombs or nudity, nothing at all like the real deal!).

So with my glass of beer in hand and still on a high from my girls night out, I settle in to picking which season I want to watch and I naturally choose the one where Samantha discovers that she has breast cancer. Now that I know what breast cancer is about, I thought it would be an interesting new way to view the show that I've seen a hundred times.

And I also couldn't help but wonder,since I know these characters so well, am I now a Samantha?

I end up watching 5 (!) episodes of Samantha discovering she has cancer, fighting her way into the best oncologist's office, dealing with hair loss, and eventually accepting her disease. Wow, can I relate. Watching these episodes, two scenes really stood out to me. The first one is of her and Carrie at a wig shop right before there was any significant hair loss and she was just trying to look and live normally – "I don't have cancer, I have a premier!" she tells the wig shop owner. This stood out because no matter how much you try to live normally (my doctor tells me to do this all the time), you still DO have cancer and nothing feels "normal" anymore. She was still trying to hold on to her old life by looking the part and I completely know that feeling. The second scene was when she was making a speech at a benefit and became overheated in her wig. She finally sweated so much she said F*#% it, and took it off to show her chemo head, inspiring the other women in the crowd to do the same. Now I know that scene was set up as a feel-good, hold your head high in the face of disease kinda moment. But I saw it as Samantha accepting that her cancer HAS changed her and her life and she just has to live with that. And live POSITIVELY with it, Samantha style – wearing pink wigs, having popsicle parties during chemo with her girlfriends, and still dating hottie Smith Jarod who shaved his head for her! As I watched her transformation from old Samantha to new Samantha, I cried and I have to admit, I finally, truly and wholly, accepted this disease in my life too.

I am a cancer patient. I am a fighter. I am a positive thinker with an army of support. So, yes, I am a Samantha.

It's Positively Cancer
March 30, 2012
Hey, look! They finally made me as a Barbie! (It's about time!)
Beautiful and Bald Barbie! Let's see if we can get it made
We did it! We WILL see a Beautiful and Bald "friend of Barbie" made to help young girls who live with hair loss due to cancer treatments, Alopecia or Trichotillomania . Also, for young girls who are having trouble coping with their mother's hair loss from chemo.

It's Positively Cancer
April 2, 2012

In the spirit of "keeping it real" when it comes to documenting my breast cancer experience, I have decided to write about some things in order not to forget them. The little details, I guess, that can get lost in the big picture, but really can be just as important to remember after I win this war and look back on the months I spent fighting it. I know that it won't be the fondest of memories, but the small, day-to-day, I'm-living-with-cancer details will make it real to me again. (And truthfully, I find some of this whole experience weird in a "I have to laugh at this!" kinda way, so I want to remember those moments!) So here it goes.

Taking A Shower.

Taking a shower for any Mom with a baby is a luxury. I usually rush through it, hoping and praying that he will just nap long enough to get the job done and that I will come out smelling clean and not like spit-up. I have been doing this shower routine since he was born. A long shower is now something that I yearn for – a time to pamper myself with all the girlie, flowery smelling shampoos and body washes, letting myself take my time to let the warm water massage my aching shoulders, taking care of the shaving rituals that us ladies have to keep ourselves beautiful, and finally stepping out into the sauna of a bathroom with the calmness and relaxation that only a great, 15 minute shower can give you. Ahhhhhhhhh………Unfortunately, those days are few and far between now that there is a baby who demands attention. My showers are fine and about 5 minutes, but far from the 15 minutes of bliss that I used to know.

Now let's fast track to the last 2 months.

I knew that chemo was going to take the hair on my head and obviously I got cool with that. (If it didn't, I got some bad chemo and it is not doing its job!) They also told me that I may lose other hair on my body as well, and, well, I just wanted to wait and see what that was all about. Guess what happens? Once you shave it, it is gone. Yup, just like the hair on my head, anything I shave doesn't grow back. Crazy. I haven't shaved my legs in 2 months (what?!). Not that I'm complaining…..too much. It is just weird. It's all gone and I have no clue when it will come back. This is some wild stuff, seriously.

So now, not only do I not have any hair to wash, but now I have nothing to shave either. My showers have gone from luxurious to functional to BORING! I have nothing to do. I don't know WHAT to do. I literally just stand there, trying to make it last as long as I can, but I am clueless about what kind of hair-free shower to take. Just. Stand. There. I can't even seem to pamper myself a little, since pampering in the past included shaving and shampooing. And the craziest part of it all is that I get out of the shower feeling like a dude. A clean dude, but not quite the lavender-smelling, freshly shaven girl I used to be. Frankly, showers have not only become bewildering, but a bit disappointing. Cancer has not only changed my life, it has changed my womanly shower ritual.

I think the hardest thing to wrap my head around is that part of me that wants to hold on to as much of my femininity as possible in the face of losing my hair and eventually a breast, and shaving my legs is part of it. And that is gone now too.

It's all good, though. A temporary glitch in the grand scheme of things. I can just see myself reading this in a couple of years and laugh, thinking "I can't believe I was so put off by not having to shave my legs every day!". But I'm telling you, when this is all over, I am taking the LONGEST shower in the most LUXURIOUS bathroom I can find, and I am going to shampoo and shave myself silly with the most expensive soaps I can get my hands on! What a glorious 20 minutes that will be!

It's Positively Cancer
April 10, 2012

This is what Chemo looks like…..it's not so scary

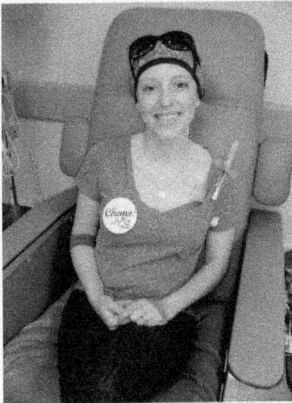

It's Positively Cancer
April 12, 2012

The most frequently asked question that I get about my breast cancer, aside from "How are you feeling?", is "How did you find it?" I have realized that in my pursuit of documenting my cancer journey, I have failed to write about the one thing that I get asked about the most and the one thing I should have on record if I want to bring awareness to other women who read this. So, here is that story.

I had been breast-feeding Charlie since he was born and around his 5 ½ month birthday I developed swelling under my right armpit. It was very uncomfortable to sleep on and after a few days, I called my OB-GYN office to ask about it. We all thought it may just be a clogged milk duct (as they were want to do to me from time to time) and to give it a week with warm compresses to see if the swelling went down. It didn't, so I went into her office…..alone……. a week and 2 days after I called. After an exam, my doctor sent me down a floor to get an ultrasound on that side to "check it out". I knew that wasn't good. The ultrasound technician was quiet and when she was done, she sent me BACK up to my doctor's office again. Now I knew this REALLY wasn't good, especially when I walk in the door and the receptionist looked up and immediately said "Mrs. Hamilton? You can go right in." Oh. Dear. God. What is going on?! My doctor sat me down and said there was a mass in the ultrasound picture and she wanted me to see a surgeon about getting a biopsy done on it. Wait a minute............I just came in here for a clogged milk duct. What are we saying here?! I stood before a nurse who was making a few phone calls, leaning against the counter and trying to keep my head on straight. But I could hear the urgency in my doctor's voice as she was telling the nurse to tell whoever was on the other line that it is a mass and I need to get in there tomorrow. All I could do was focus on the kindness of the nurse who was dealing with me and plaster a it's-going-to-be-nothing fake smile on my face.

I see the surgeon the next day and we set up the biopsy for the following Tuesday, about 5 days later. I get the result the next day by phone (which my surgeon has apologized for) saying that there are cancer cells in the mass and in a lymph node, which was the swollen part under my arm which started this process. Within the next week, I had a PET scan, CAT scan, met my oncologist to find out I have Stage III cancer, underwent out-patient surgery to put a port-a-cath in, and started my first chemo regimen. By Charlie's 6 month birthday, cancer was in my life. Just like that. Amazing.

So there is my story. And here is my soap-box speech – LADIES, check your self and report anything weird to your doctor. This isn't meant to scare, just inform. My hope is to share my story to keep the ladies out there healthy and happy! (And please, for the love of God, don't read anything online about cancer – There is some scary shit out there!)

It's Positively Cancer
April 15, 2012
I told you all that I'd do it – GO PREDS!

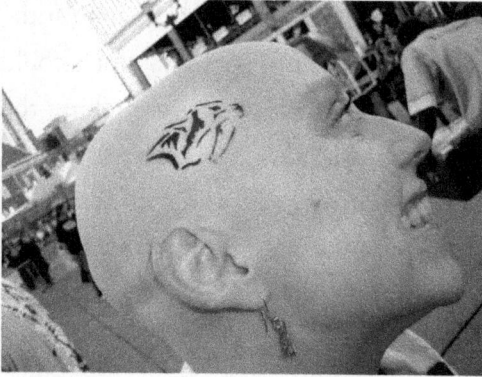

It's Positively Cancer
April 20, 2012
A couple of chemo treatments ago, my nurse informed me that my red blood count was low and that I needed to relax and rest more. To "stop working" was exactly what she told me…..yeah, right! That just can't happen, so Jesse and I found a good compromise – he and the other managers would take over at the Pub and I would scale back to once a week, leaving me with time to complete my other job as Festival Director for a local festival happening in May without the added stress of daily Pub operations. So now I am at home more, doing most of my festival work over the phone or via email and spending most of my days with Charlie. And in my homebody mode of life, I have discovered entertainment in

a great cable channel called RetroHD that plays old movies all day every day – I'm talking westerns, Hitchcock, 80s comedies, you name it. But most importantly, this channel is not afraid to also feature A MUSICAL.

Now on my side of the family, musicals are as familiar to us as hockey is to Canada. Us Smiths have seen them all and can sing more songs from them than what should be considered normal. (There is a bit of family connection with the genre; I have a great-uncle who was Fred Astaire's choreographer – no joke – so we've always had a soft spot for musicals.) My grandfather was famous at family gatherings for starting sing-a-longs with a resounding "OHHHHHHHH............!" and then marching straight into a gleeful rendition of "76 Trombones Led the Big Parade" from The Music Man. I grew up on musicals as a kid and have seen all the classics, some of them over and over again. My sisters and I would even dance out some numbers, like the barn-raising scene from Seven Brides for Seven Brothers or just snapping our fingers Jets-style down the hallway of our home mimicking West Side Story. When I hear any song from Singing in the Rain, The Sound of Music, or The Music Man, I get a warm blanket feeling of familiarity around my heart and want to sing that song from the tops of a mountain like Maria does.

I know it isn't very cool of me to nerd out to musicals when maybe I should be rediscovering my old Nirvana or Alice In Chains CDs instead for a music outlet. I have seen the look on Jesse's face when I start singing some random song around the house from a musical he's never heard of, much less seen. (Charlie, however, absolutely loves my rendition of "The Farmer and the Cowman Should Be Friends" from Oklahoma or "Happy Talk" from South Pacific – they are great kids songs, at least the way I do it!) But music is about bringing happiness and joy to people and those songs can do that for me. Besides, music is also healing, whether it is from heart-break, loss, or any other malady. It lifts you up, brings you peace, and even makes you laugh. So maybe musicals will actually help me heal and deal with cancer too, not only by filling my "restful" days at home with a bit of throw-back entertainment, but also by bringing around wonderful memories and laughter as I begin to pass my musical-loving torch on to (poor) Charlie.

And how can one NOT keep their spirits uplifted, their attitude positive, and seriously keep themselves from smiling when they have THIS song stuck in their head…..
I Love To Laugh Sing Along (from Mary Poppins)

It's Positively Cancer
April 21, 2012

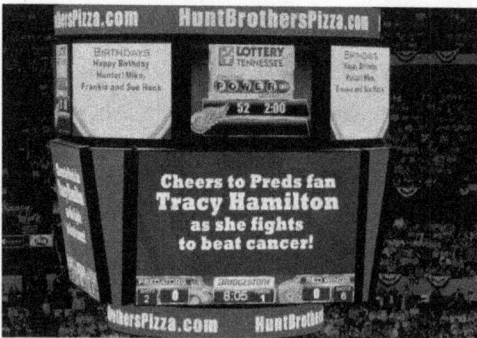

I made the JUMBOTRON at the Preds Playoff Game last night!
SO COOL!!! Thank you to everyone who was involved in surprising me – you picked a great game for it (2nd Round!)!!
You guys ROCK!

It's Positively Cancer
April 25, 2012

Charlie's Angels

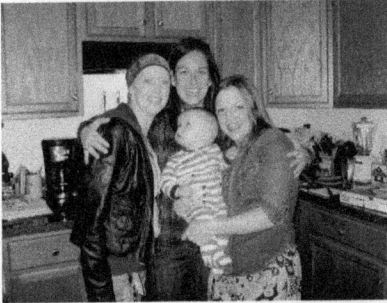

My sister Rosemary (*middle*)came to town from Portland, Oregon to surprise me with a visit! YAY –
second surprise of the week for me, I am so blessed!

It's Positively Cancer
April 28, 2012

I know some of you have been asking if there is anything I need or anything you can do during this whole cancer journey, and I think that I have found something that actually might be both fun AND helpful! If you can believe it, I am the Festival Director for the Riverside Blossom Festival in East Nashville and have been organizing it for months now. It is a neighborhood street fair complete with 2 music stages, craft beer, food, and family activities (we even have a BOUNCY CASTLE!!! Sweet!). It is taking place Saturday May 12th (2 weeks away ...... AHHHHHH!!!!!) and what I am lacking are some volunteers to help that day. We need people to help get the vendors in the right spot, parking, get the musicians what they need, set-up and general maintenance in the beer "tent" area, check IDs during the festival, clean-up, and help with the kids activities.

Anyone interested? ....there may be a T-shirt involved! If you are, let me know. It would be extremely helpful and I would greatly appreciate it – I promise it will be fun too! Don't sweat it if you can't, but definitely come to the festival anyway! Did I mention there is BEER there? I did? AND a Bouncy Castle?! Okay...I know I've definitely tempted some of you! Thanks and check it out at www.riversideblossomfest.com or the FB page!

It's Positively Cancer
May 2, 2012

"You just gotta keep livin' man, L-I-V-I-N."

I have been thinking of this quote lately. These are words spoken by the great Wooderson (Matthew McConaughey in a role he was born to play) in the cult classic "Dazed and Confused", a movie that is on my list of "5 movies I would take with me to a deserted island". I just love how he delivers this line in his older stoner, Southern drawl and to me, this line summed up the whole movie. The kids were celebrating the last day of school and living in the moment, as teenagers are want to do. They don't want to think about the future, they want to live in the present. Granted, living in the present to them is smoking pot on the 50 yard line, hazing incoming freshman, and going to a party at the moon tower, but that is exactly what you want to do in high school – ENJOY LIFE, even if it meant breaking the rules a bit.

I guess I've been thinking about this quote for a number of reasons. One could be because I am fighting cancer to keep livin'. Heavy, I know, but that is exactly what I am doing. It could also be because my doctors have basically told me to keep living my life, especially during the chemo treatments. From the moment I started the treatment process, they have been very vocal about keeping my daily routine as normal as possible, without over exerting myself, of course. They have said that they will make my life as comfortable as they can and before I know it, this will all be just something I did or something I went through – like my pregnancy with Charlie, or that time when I was dumped by a boyfriend on the phone (so WRONG!) but then found my independence and voice as a single gal, or those crazy-busy Sunday nights I worked at the Boundr'y and Virago with my bartender buddy Jimbo. Soon, cancer will all be a memory, with just as big of an impact as those memories, and I can then say I lived through that (too!).

But I think the real reason this quote comes to mind for

me is because I DO want to keep livin', but in a way that is different than how I used to live. While I have been planning for the future by making the Pub as successful as possible and securing my family financially, emotionally, and physically and will always continue to do so, I want to start living in the present more. Charlie does it every day and there is something to be learned by that. I'm not saying that I want to party at the moon tower every night (even though every once in a while wouldn't be bad!), but I want to try to do things now that will make my life enjoyable and worth the journey. And the key is not to be afraid to live. To really do the things I have put off AND to do the things that come to mind the minute they come. To do at least one enjoyable thing every single day, whether that means treating myself to cheesecake or a really delicious IPA beer, or taking Charlie to the zoo or Adventure Science Museum, or even daydreaming about the vacation Jesse and I are going to take when I am better. Wooderson is right, man – you gotta keep on livin', ya'll, and I want to do it thinking like a teenager while acting like an adult.........well, most of the time!

(And just in case you were wondering, the other 4 movies are "Goodfellas", "Finding Nemo", "Star Wars: Return of the Jedi" before George Lucas effed it up, and my all-time favorite movie to quote, "The Princess Bride". Now, how would I find a TV/DVD player to play them on or electricity on this deserted island.........?)

It's Positively Cancer
May 17, 2012

Guess who has a smattering of blond peach fuzz on top of her head?......and guess who's going to wash it?!

It's Positively Cancer
May 19, 2012

A few nights ago, I worked an event at the Tennessee State Museum for our special event bartending services business, Hamilton Bartending Services. HBS is the mother company to the Village Pub of sorts – Jesse and I got it going in 2005 bartending mostly weddings, art shows, and private parties. We would pack up our 1993 AroStar minivan with coolers of ice, mixes, barware, and sometimes even a portable bar and drive it in our service tuxedos to various event spaces, farms, businesses, and wedding venues across Middle Tennessee. It has proven to be a lot of work, but a lot of fun over the years and we have grown it immensely. We now even rent glassware and hire other bartenders to help us out. Being that my name is "on the door" so to speak, I don't do as many events as I used to in order to give our other employees more work, so it has become a rare and fun treat to for me when I go out to work an event and I really enjoy myself.

This was the first event I have worked since my diagnosis and I must admit to being somewhat nervous. Can I still do it? Will my energy wane? Can I keep up the pace of a party without needing a break and feeling like a slacker? And, what about my bald head.....how does THAT look with a tuxedo on? Professional? Cancer-patienty? Unprofessional? Luckily, the TN State Museum is a long-time client and their events are short, so I gave myself a break and tried not to worry about it. So, after checking my appearance with Jesse a dozen times ("Are you SURE this hat doesn't look stupid? Do I look sick now that I have no eyelashes? If I wear a little lipstick, will that help me look more professional?"), I was on my way downtown.

As it turns out, this was no ordinary art show that we usually bartend for the museum. The artist for this show is none other than John Mellencamp (apparently he is now painting the little houses pink instead of just singing about them – who knew?!) and it was a BIG DEAL for the museum. I'm talking a VIP bar for him and his famous friends separate from the main gallery bar, 3 bartenders and 4 servers from us instead of the usual 2 bartenders only, and they added liquor to the menu of beer and wine and a big fancy food spread with a cake bearing JM's name. Us lowly service workers even got a speech from the head museum ladies about how we need to fade into the background, do NOT take pictures or ask for autographs, and if there is ANY mention of what went on in the VIP bar in the Enquirer Magazine (!?) she will know that it was one of us who leaked it. I am not kidding – she actually said that. They also expected to have around 400-500 people show up for it, press included, and everyone was going to want as many drinks as they could get in the 2 hours or so we were pouring. Game On.

Needless to say, once the party started, I had no time to

think about my hat or my lipstick. I was working the floor like a mad woman, making sure guests got drinks, both bars had plenty of ice, the food was in place at both areas, the cocktail tables were bussed, and the museum ladies were happy. I could only manage a quick smile at Meg Ryan (so cool!!) as we passed each other in the hall. But after a while as things got into a steady pace, I was able to get a good look around and I started to really notice all the ladies dressed up and dolled out for this event. Most were very stylish and well-put together and I started to feel self-conscious again. To make matters worse, I stopped in the ladies room to wash my hands and there was a full-length mirror. Ugh. I am usually all about holding my (bald) head high and not caring, but something just hit me. I felt right then like I was the only one in the whole world with cancer and EVERYONE knew because I just couldn't hide it and they were all staring. And then I felt myself get teary – not a sad teary, but a mad one. WHY ME?! I just want to look normal, feel normal, BE normal and that is not at all what I am right now. Damn it, I am tired of thinking about cancer, living with cancer, talking about cancer – I just want my life back to NORMAL!!!!!

But the fact of the matter is that it will never be normal again. And after I collected myself and resumed my duties at the party, I realized that it is okay to get mad every once in a while about that. Cancer pisses me off and I have every right to be upset and angry. Besides, the angrier I get at cancer, the more I am determined to beat it once and for all (I have a terrible reputation of letting anger become a spark to ignite a determination to win, just ask my high school track coach!). Life will become cancer-free normal soon and I know that. I just want it to get here already.

When the event was over and we were loading up our van, I had taken my hat off because I was hot and placed it in my back pocket. One of the quieter museum ladies noticed and asked me if I had cancer. When I told her yes, she said she did too and was 6 years in remission. She was back to her normal. She gave me a bright smile, shook her lovely red curls, and wished me good health and luck as she returned to the after-party. It gave me hope that soon my after-party will also be just around the corner.

It's Positively Cancer changed their cover photo.
May 20, 2012

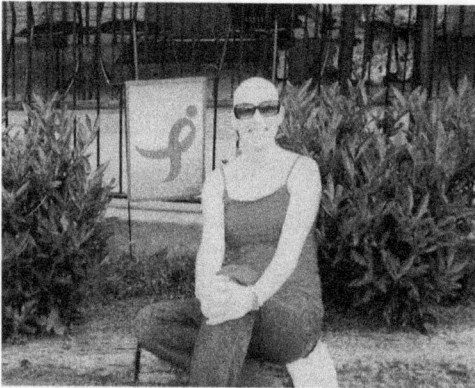

That's Me in front of the Pub!

It's Positively Cancer

May 24, 2012

Check this out ya'll! I've been invited to speak this weekend in a panel for cancer survivors / fighters at a conference called Creativity Moves Nashville, which is all about giving back to your community through creative means. Cool, huh?! Here's their website with my picture and short bio http://creativitymoves.com/cancer-survivors

Wish me luck – I don't know how great of a public speaker I am going to be, but I will give it a try anyway!

It's Positively Cancer

May 27, 2012

Here is why I love living in East Nashville:

I was working at the Pub last night and talking to some regulars out on the porch. Being that it was a hot summer evening, it was too warm to wear a hat and I was flying the bald flag. We were talking about the heat and our "summer do's" and how great and easy it is to not have hair when you sweat so much (I was talking to 2 guys, both of which have closely shaved heads). One of them looks at me as asks, "So, what prompted you to shave your head?" I was a bit taken aback – I figured by now most people knew what was going on (especially since we were standing near the Breast Cancer Awareness flag that is in front of the Pub). Nope. He thought I did it on my own; cool-kid, hipster style. When I said,

"Breast Cancer made me do it", I think I gave him the last answer he ever thought he would hear.

Ahhhhh, East Nashville – a place where bald women are normal, accepted, and not assumed to have cancer!

It's Positively Cancer
May 30, 2012

It was a GREAT EVENT on Sunday afternoon at Creativity Moves Nashville at Belmont! Thank you to Jacob Weiss for inviting me to speak – I enjoyed everyone who participated and you guys put on a great juggling show! This is a picture of our songwriting team ...... together we wrote a song called "Spreading Smiles"! Stay tuned for the lyrics when I can get a hold of them, ya'll – it's a Grammy in the making (or a least a good country song – move over Martina McBride!)!

Great meeting and talking with you today at Creativity Moves Nashville. Look forward to seeing you at the Pub!

It's Positively Cancer
June 8, 2012

Status Update:

I have ONE MORE CHEMO TREATMENT left – Whoo Hoo!!!!

After 8 weeks of every other week, hardcore, makes-your-hair-fall-out chemo followed by 12 weeks of lighter but more routine, only-your-eyelashes-fall-out (?!) treatment, this Tuesday June 12th will mark the end of a huge stage of this whole damn process that I can thankfully say is behind me!! And the best part is, aside from a few doctor appointments, I will have a blessed 4 weeks of nothing-cancer related until my surgery......it's a cancer vacation!

So guess what I have planned?.......

A Tour Of Pleasures.

This lady plans to do it up Eat Pray Love style. I want to have a few awesome meals along the lines of Sole Mio downtown or Eastland Cafe right down the street. Then I hope to really spoil my son with my extra energy boost by going to Radnor Lake and exploring a new park with him. THEN.....well, the love part has nothing to do with ya'll!

Yes, 4 weeks of remembering why you fight to begin with — to live your life to the fullest. What a great way to re-energize yourself to fight the second half of the battle, right?

And since this is an update, it looks like the surgery.....which will be a double mastectomy to make sure there is NO CHANCE of reoccurrence......will be about mid-July. And that is cool by me.

It's Positively Cancer

June 13, 2012

Bummer News:

I go into the chemo office yesterday for my last treatment armed with cupcakes for the nurses, a celebratory attitude,.......aaand apparently a 102.5 temperature. It turns out that my crazy night sweats and freakishly dramatic chills I had the night before were not from chemo and anxiety.

I have an infection of some sorts (results to be determined later). So now I have to skip this week's chemo treatment in order to take ($100!) antibiotics for 7 days to rid myself of whatever it turns out to be.

Really, cancer? Really? On my LAST FREAKING DAY of chemo?! Not 2 weeks ago, not 2 months ago, not even tomorrow! Sigh.

I know this whole cancer experience is a bunch of little tests of will and strength sometimes, but this one was a big disappointment. But what are you going to do? I guess buy more cupcakes and proclaim June 19th instead as a milestone day.

Thanks for all the encouragement and excitement from those who wanted to celebrate with me yesterday. Keep some of that bottled and we will pop that cork again next week!

It's Positively Cancer
June 20, 2012
Drumroll please............

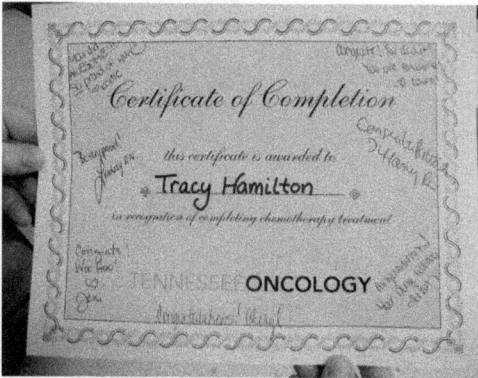

It is official! Chemo is OVER!!!!!!!!!!!

After a week of full of trials – fighting this infection, 2 days of a warm 85 degree house as we fixed our broken air conditioner, and having to put our beloved 16 year old cat Sam down (so sad) – we finally have something to celebrate! The staff was really great too. On your last day in the chemo room, the nurses make a big announcement to everyone there that it is your final treatment and then let you ring a very LOUD gong as if to say "in your face, cancer!" I was even presented a Certificate of Completion signed by all the nurses, which of course is now framed and hung up where I can see it every day to remind myself that I CAN DO THIS!

Whewwww, what a relief! Now my hair and eyelashes have a chance to grow back (I do have a healthy growth of red fuzz on my head already!) and I will have until the end of July free of weekly appointments, hooray! I almost don't know what to do with myself........oh, who am I kidding! I will live it up, which means I will live blissfully NORMAL for a while! It'll be a nice break and a chance to prepare for the next fight.

It's Positively Cancer

June 23, 2012 (A Preds hat and NHL Hockey puck signed by Jordan Tootoo)

My sister Kelly surprised me yesterday with this (apparently, she has very cool connections!)! Rumor has it that he has also read some of my Predators posts on this page, how awesome is that? I am now a bonafide TooToo fan for life .... not that that was a stretch for me, I DO own a TooToo jersey! It just goes to show what a big heart he has to go with his big personality that he took the time to write something encouraging for little 'ole me. Thanks Kelly and GO PREDS!

It's Positively Cancer
June 26, 2012

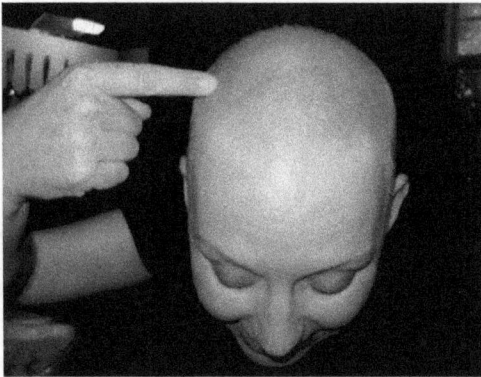

Look What's Growing!!

It's Positively Cancer
July 2, 2012

I can't wait to join the ranks with this AWESOME girl – I will be with good company!

This little girl deserves as many likes and shares as possible. (Special thanks to the Twitterverse for passing this photo on to us) Stupid Cancer indeed. (Posted picture of young bald girl holding a sign saying 'Stupid Cancer')

It's Positively Cancer
July 7, 2012

Ever since Charlie was born and I have been more of a homebody, I listen and have become addicted to NPR. I've always listened here and there in the past, but now it is a constant in my daily routine. Programs with clever names like "All Things Considered" and "Fresh Air" got me hooked into listening to the station because I was always guaranteed to hear something interesting and current without being bored to death. I have heard some really cool interviews with Alec Baldwin, Hugh Laurie, and Nora Ephron. Science Fridays always seem to open my mind to things I would never think about, like why tomatoes grow the way they do and the "God Cell". And don't get me started on "Car Talk" – I love, love, LOVE those guys and I was crushed to hear that they retired from their show.

So the other day I was listening to a program on "Talk of the Nation" about honesty and how often people lie. It was fascinating – they did experiments asking people to solve as many math problems as they could in 5 minutes and for each problem they got right, they would get paid $1. The twist was that when the 5 minutes were up, each person counted up their own correct answers, then they would shred their paper in a paper shedder before reporting to the experimenter to tell them how many they got right. What they didn't know was that the paper shredder only shredded the sides of the paper, leaving the main portion intact to collect for accuracy. They found that on average each person would report say 6 correct answers, but really had gotten only 4 right. The conclusion? Many people lie a little bit if they think the stakes aren't that high.

I guess I found it fascinating because it made me think about how honest I am. In general, I think I fair pretty well. And to prove it…….. my true weight right now is 132 pounds (at last doctor's appointment); I claim to have been a vegetarian since I was 18 years old but I had eaten chicken a handful of times in those first few years; and, even though I was a CHAMP at the game "Heads Up, 7 Up!" when I was a kid, it was only because I cheated by looking at the shoes of the kid who tapped me. Whewwwww……I'm glad I got that off my chest!

But when I started to think about it, how honest am I REALLY, especially to myself. Are there parts of my life that I should've handled better than I think I did? Sure. Am I more of a bitch at times rather than this sunny, look-on-the-bright-side kind of gal that I like to think I am? Absolutely. This whole cancer experience has worked wonders on self-imposed reality checks for sure. But after turning off the radio and putting Charlie down for his nap, I started really thinking about my life and being honest about it. This can bring you to a crazy dark place if you aren't careful, let me tell you. I say that only because I started to be really honest with myself about my diagnosis. I think staying positive is a wonderful thing and necessary when fighting cancer to give yourself hope and a chance to live. But, there is also a hard reality to be honest about. Like, no matter how great things are going with my treatments so far, cancer can still spread. Like, I can go through chemo, surgery, and radiation and cancer can still come back. Like, cancer can still kill me. See.....pretty scary stuff. But it is true. It has now sunk in how wonderful a word REMISSION is.

The truth is, as I was sitting on the couch thinking about all this as I was trying to choke down lunch and not freak out, I realized that even though the outlook can be frightening, I still have a great chance of coming out a winner. My hair is already growing back and my tumor, which I used to be able to feel pretty well, has now shrunk to the point of being harder to find. I even saw my surgeon smile after examining me a couple of weeks ago (which she has not done yet so far to me – she is VERY businesslike), which gave me a boost of confidence that the treatments are working well. So, I have decided that even though I am glad I was honest with myself about the scary side of cancer, I am not going to go down that road again in my brain.

Maybe I'll take a break from NPR a bit too. Charlie should listen to something else anyway and I have a mean Nirvana CD collection that I could introduce him to. I mean, honestly, isn't that more fun?

It's Positively Cancer
July 14, 2012

CANCERCATION!

Whoo-Hoo! An honest-to-goodness, let's get out of dodge for a few days trek to the woods to rest up for the second stage of treatment. I highly recommend David Crockett (yes David, not Davy) State Park – lots of hiking, fishing, and paddle boating!......or if you are like us and get rained on the whole 4 days, lots of movies, food, and beer! YAY!

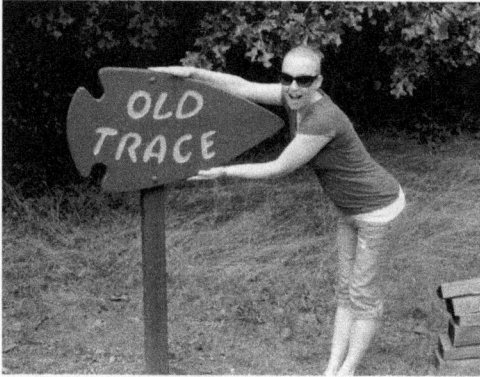

It's Positively Cancer
July 18, 2012
It was a party!

This past Sunday, me and a few girlfriends got together for a "Girls Night Out", with special attention paid to our "girls", at the Urban Grub in the 12 South District (this is my special shout-out to my friends who are running the place – Jimbo and Garth, it was so great to see you and your success!). I figured I should take my boobs out for drinks and (apparently) a little fondling before the surgery on the 31st takes them away. So off we were for a night of many drinks, wonderful food, and wild girl conversations that could only be had when you sit 15 women at a table – that may or may not have met one another – and just let them loose!

I can only speak for myself, but I had a great time and I was so happy to see the table of women sitting there, each representing a different part of my life. I have always thought that I am more of a boy's friend than a girl's friend – I can be quite a tomboy if you let me, sports are kinda my thang, and I have just always found talking to guys easier for some reason. I guess all my years of bartending trained me to be cool around the boys because that was who I mostly waited on. I have to admit how surprised I was at myself for not only having more girlfriends than I thought, but for having such GREAT ones! (Why don't I hang out with them more?...this will be remedied!) Every lady sitting there has such a strong will and a wonderful heart – I am truly blessed to call them friends. Looking around at their beautiful faces throughout the night made me glad to know them and even more glad to STILL know them.

I cannot thank cancer for much, but I have to admit that it had brought us all together and I am grateful for that. I am also grateful for which ever friend it was that actually put her hand down my dress and gave the "girls" a night to remember....what are friends for, right?

It's Positively Cancer
July 29, 2012

The countdown is on…..I have 2 days until surgery, 2 days left with the girls before they are replaced with newer models. Tuesday July 31st at 9am is the day that I will hopefully get rid of this stupid cancer for good. I see this surgery as getting closer to the denouement of my cancer story and everything else afterwards will (hopefully!) just tidy up all the loose ends towards a happy ending.

I have to admit, however, of being pretty nervous about this stage – the idea of "going under" scares the beejezus out of me. Granted, I have done it twice before (wisdom teeth and when I got my port put in) and I had Charlie via C-Section (which I was awake for, for crying out loud!) But…..this seems bigger and scarier. I am already getting butterflies in my stomach, my nails are chewed down to nubs, and I find myself wanting to "say good-bye" to people I won't see for a couple of weeks (what?!). I am driving myself a little crazy and now I just want it to be over with.

But then I was in Charlie's room looking for a book to read to him and I spotted my collection of Harry Potter books that sit nicely on the top shelf of his bookshelf. Then it dawns on me…..July 31st is Harry Potter's birthday.

To some, it is no big surprise that I know when Harry Potter's birthday is, but for those who don't, allow me to explain. I am a Potterhead. I admit it. I not only have every copy of the books (which I have read a least 5 times EACH), but I have them in both hardback and paperback. I own the movies, have a couple of T-shirts, and there are 2 canvas book cover prints hanging on the wall in Charlie's room. I have also been known to BE Harry Potter for Halloween (twice!) and wear a charm of a Hippogriff on a necklace from time to time. And, yes, I am also a 35 year old grown-up. And apparently a dork.

So when I realize this significance, I started thinking about how the Harry Potter series plot line is kinda like fighting cancer (here's where I'll get REALLY dorky on you). At first, Voldemort....or cancer ...is just lying under the surface, weak and powerless, waiting to gain strength to rise up and take over. Harry Potter...or me, in this scenario... may or may not really know of his existence, but he is there. Then after a few signs here or there, he finally shows his ugly, snakelike head and it is scary. You know he's killed others and now he is after you. At first you, your family, and your friends are in denial and disbelief. But soon, there is no denying the fact that he is big, he is real, and he is taking over. The urge is there to run and hide, but you know that eventually you have to turn around and fight, knowing also that you may die, but deciding that in the end you did everything in your power to defeat him. As the plot comes to an end ....in the books, at least....it is Harry Potter who emerges victorious and Voldemort ultimately meets his demise.

As geeky as that may sound, I found some solace in this comparison. Bravery is an ongoing theme throughout the book series and it is what made our heroes persevere with every challenge that they faced. It is what made them Gryffindors. Being a Gryffindork, it calms me to think that all I need is bravery to beat my Voldemort. So instead of being scared when I am up against this monster, I need to face it, endure it, and know that I am doing everything I can to defeat this evil in my world.

To be the GIRL who lived.

I guess it is time to crack open Book #1 again. Maybe I will take the first 2 books with me to the hospital, just in case I need an extra jolt of inspiration.

4

My Daughter My Best Friend II

I well remember the day she called to tell me she had cancer. It really wasn't much of a conversation. I always thought of Tracy as a female me – laid-back, easy-going, emotionally level headed – so it wasn't a very emotionally charged call.

"Hey, Pops, I just wanted to let you know that I just came from the Doctor and it looks like I have stage three breast cancer."

That's what I loved about Tracy. She wasn't much for chit-chatty phone conversations. She got to the point and just put it out there. Then she'd give it a minute to sink in.

"Oh ...... okay ..... well, I'm sure the doctors know what they are doing, so if you just follow their instructions, I'm sure this will just be another bump in the road for ya."

She agreed and the rest of the conversation was just going over the details and schedules and letting her know that I'm there for her and Jesse for whatever they need.

That's the problem with cancer nowadays. You see so

many stories of people who are diagnosed with cancer and a year later they talk about how these people are cancer survivors as if they had a hang nail.

It's like the Apollo program at NASA back a bit in my youth. We all remember every moment of the first time we landed a man on the Moon, but after a while, it became almost an afterthought on the evening news... "Oh and we'll leave you tonight with a photo of a couple of our astronauts playing a round of golf on the surface of the Moon."

One of the hardest feelings I had to deal with after her passing was the feeling of how casual I responded to her along the way. The guilt of not taking it serious enough can way heavy on a Dads heart. Did I give her reason to feel alone in this battle? Did my reactions to her make her feel frustrated or that her own Dad wasn't that concerned that his daughter was DYING? How could I move on in my life feeling that my daughter had passed away without her Dad showing up emotionally?

This is the one person who was with her every step of her life. I was the first one she set her eyes on when she was born. I was the one who took her to the beach all those times when her baby sister needed a quiet nap time. I was the one who went to every swim meet, track meet and every activity she was involved with during her youth. I was the one who was sitting at the bar of every restaurant and bar she worked in throughout her career at least once a week – without fail.

This girl lived thirty seven years and if you added up the weeks she went without seeing her Dad, I'm guessing it would not add up to a year. I was always a part of Tracy's life and it was NEVER out of any obligation – I wanted to be there. I enjoyed being around her. It was always the best day of my week.

How could I possibly live with myself feeling that I was complacent during the final chapters of her life? No big deal, kiddo, just deal with it and you'll be fine.

But I refused to beat myself up over these feelings for a couple of reasons.

First, I knew that I was not the only one who felt that way. If you could go back and read the comments on her facebook page, you'd see that everyone who knew Tracy had the same attitude. Cancer didn't have a chance against this girl. In the early stages, there was almost a humorous feel to all the posts and comments. If anybody can beat cancer, Tracy was a sure bet! Everyone I talked to had the same feeling that there would be a time after all this that we would be celebrating how Tracy's attitude and approach to life really kicked the butt of cancer.

There was not one person who knew Tracy that would have guessed that the story would go the way it did. Not…. One…. Person!

But a pattern quietly grew with each phone call.

"Well, Pops, I got some good news and some bad news."

The good news was never that good and the bad news was leaving me more and more speechless with a numb, fragile response of just saying, "Really?" I was beginning to dread the days she had a doctors appointment and would sink emotionally in the late afternoons when the phone rang.

The other reason I wouldn't beat myself up over the feelings of complacency is because I knew it wasn't true. Sure, when I was out in public, I always presented the most positive attitude I could generate at the time. I wasn't being phony, I was being realistic. In times of struggle, it is so important to present a positive energy at all times. It wasn't a phony energy because I truly felt the same way everyone else who knew Tracy felt. No matter how bad the odds were, I would never bet against Tracy. In fact, the more the odds were against Tracy, the more she liked it.

I remember when she was in high school and she was the track star in the long distance races. She loved her coach Brown and she loved to run.

It was one of the important track meets of the year – one of the state qualifiers – and I noticed that coach Brown was spending a lot of time encouraging one of the other girls and barely talking to Tracy. When we took our seats in the stand – being a state qualifier, the coaches had to be in the stands when the races began – I brought it up to coach Brown.

He just looked at me and smiled.

" The other girl is kind of a whiner who needs a lot of pampering and encouragement to run well. Tracy doesn't really like her too much and it pisses her off when I show more attention to her and not Tracy. I get the best out of both runners by doing that"

Sure enough, as the race evolved, it was clear that Tracy

and the other girl were oblivious to the rest of the pack … it was one against the other in their world. When they got to last lap of the race, Tracy put on the after burners and left that poor other girl coughing up dust for the next several weeks. As she was gathering her breath afterwards, she made several glaring looks up at coach Brown and I. Thankfully, this time, those looks were directed at coach Brown and not me.

"Well, I gotta go coddle the other one… you give Tracy a big hug for me …. I'm sure she won't be talking to me for a couple of days now."

That was Tracy.

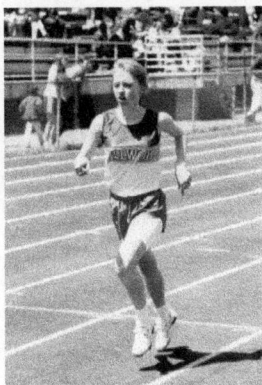

There was another time when I was working in the music business at BMI. We had our annual Christmas lunch/party at a fancy hotel ballroom less than a block from a bar Tracy bartended. I wasn't much of a corporate guy, so I was more than happy to bail from the festivities at the earliest time I could without getting into hot water with the brass and go hang with Tracy.

When I got there and made myself comfortable at the bar while Tracy fixed my drink, I told her that I told a bunch of the co-workers that I was coming here and if they got tired of the corporate nonsense, they were welcome to join me .... but I didn't think there would be more than a couple of takers to my invite.

By five o'clock that afternoon, the bar was packed literally standing room only – even a hand full of those corporate directors I was so afraid of getting in hot water for leaving early! Poor Tracy was the only bartender slinging drinks. I was stuck in the far corner of the bar drinking my Jack'n Cokes and raising my glass to her with an innocent, 'golly-gee-look-at-all-these-people' smile every time she glared at me.

The next day I called her to see if she was still talking to me. She assured me that she was fine but I'd better let her know when the Christmas party is next year so she could have more staff available to work the bar. Of course being the Dad that always puts a positive spin on every disaster, I was quick to turn the topic to how much she made in tips (I was annoyingly persistent in reminding all my co-workers that I knew how much their Christmas bonus was and they damn well better tip the bartender well!). She admitted that she walked out the door with more money in her pockets than she'd ever made before.

Thankfully, it became a tradition until I retired that the BMI Christmas party always ended up at Tracy's bar. Even when she and Jesse opened their new place on the East side, I made the very same mistake – I KID YOU NOT – by telling her when I arrived early that I didn't think many would come out to the east side like they did when she was just a block away. Of course, she knew her Dad too well and just smiled with that 'sure Dad' look. Sure enough, as the afternoon grew on the Pub began to fill until the crowd was filling in the entire place inside and out in the patio, with plenty of employees on board to keep those drinks flowing.

That was Tracy too.

Everyone who knew Tracy would agree that the crazier the situation, the more Tracy excelled. That's why they called her T-Rock. Anyone who worked with her knows when the situation got a little crazy, you WANTED Tracy on your side. She could roll up her sleeves with that 'Game On' look like noone else.

That's why so many of us took her battle with cancer so lightly initially. It was hard to imagine that cancer had any chance with this girl.

It's also the reason those of us who knew her were so numb and speechless for the last six months of her life. When we all began to realize that there was a good chance this wouldn't have a happy ending, we were all absolutely overwhelmed with the sadness.

There were so many nights towards the end when I would go home and just sit alone in my living room. Numb. Tears rolling down my cheeks. Unable to respond to any thoughts. Unable to sleep. Just staring at the TV that was sometimes on, and others times off. It didn't matter. I was glad I lived alone. Each days journey sucked so much energy out of my heart that the evenings left me with only enough energy to breath. The very thought that Tracy would lose the battle to cancer was unthinkable. But it was becoming the new reality.

I remember on one chemo session I took her to she said something that truly reflected who my daughter was.

" You know Dad, I don't know if I'm going to beat cancer, but I can promise you I will never let cancer beat me."

That was my girl.

After her passing, there were so many emotions and feelings that I had to deal with. Some days I would see a picture of Tracy and it would make me smile as I gathered up so many memories that were shared with this great young lady. Some days I would see a picture of Tracy and would be overcome with a sadness in how much I have lost.

It was the same picture.

Everyone deals with a loss like this in their own way. I just smile an empty smile when people tell me they know exactly what I'm going through because they lost their Dad a few years ago. Everybody has this need to relate, I suppose. I don't want to be the poster boy for Dads who have lost their child to cancer. I didn't sign up for that. I have no desire to be looked at as the authority of Dads who have to go to a cemetery to visit their child. All I know is that this was the hand I was dealt and I will always play my hands to win. I'm not sure some days how I do it, but every time I visit Tracy's grave site, I always let her know that – ' I'm not letting cancer beat me either, kid.'

September 1st is Tracy's birthday. I never want to be around anyone on that day except Kelly and Rosemary. It's a day that reminds me that I have gone another year without my daughter and best friend.

December 15th is the day she passed away. I am happy to get with people who knew her at her Pub to have some drinks and talk about her life. Some people might find that a bit odd or backwards, but I don't. As a Dad, I never worry about any hand I've been dealt that may cause me to suffer. As long as my girls don't suffer, I'm good. December 15th is the day Tracy stopped suffering.

Any good Dad would celebrate that.

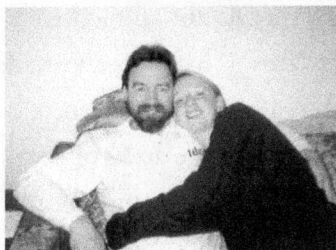

5

The Journey Continues

It's Positively Cancer

August 6, 2012

Status Update from the Island of Healing and Isolation:

First of all, I want to say THANK YOU for all the lovely cards, flowers, messages, and gifts that I have received in the past week. My home smells like a rose garden and it is truly motivating to heal quickly when I see the array of "Feel Better Soon" cards scattered about my house. I am honored to have "Dumbledore's Army" supporting me! (Yes, Harry Potter references will still keep coming…..)

As far as the surgery results, here is what we know right now. We have destroyed some of the horcruxes, but Voldemort is not quite dead yet. The good news is that they got all the cancer cells out of the breast area and the expanders have been put in. The incision sites look good and are healing nicely. I've been home since Thursday and have been resting a lot – if anyone wants to know the ins-and-outs of Olympic water polo or volleyball, let me know; I have been watching A LOT of TV at home. Jesse and I have also made it into Season 3 of "Breaking Bad" and we are addicted......pun completely intended. My family has been with me every waking minute and they have been wonderful caretakers.

However, there was some bummer news. My surgeon found more cancer cells in other lymphnodes (which they removed) and they were "alive" – meaning that they COULD HAVE the ability to spread. However, they believe that since we had started chemo so quickly, that may not be the case. Radiation treatment is next on the schedule and that should kill it for good. However, they did tell me that there may be a possibility of more chemo (sigh), depending on the results of other tests that they are running this week. I will see both my plastic surgeon and my surgeon this Thursday and Friday, respectively, and I will know more then.

But, on the bright side, it was mostly good. Charlie also turned 1 year old on Thursday and will be possibly coming home today (he has been staying with Jesse's parents so I can rest). He has discovered the wonderful world of light switches and has been getting better about drinking out of a sippy cup in my absence. It will be so AWESOME to see his sweet face and remind myself that all this treatment, surgery, and pain is so that I can be with him for many years to come and have the chance to embarrass him in front of girlfriends for liking light switches so much.

Thanks again for all the support and know that the love is coming right back to you all!

It's Positively Cancer
August 18, 2012

I find it very ironic that now that ALL my hair is growing back, I can't reach to shave what I don't want. I went from a hairless cat with chemo brain to a woolly mammoth with no boobs. Really, cancer......really?!

It's Positively Cancer
August 22, 2012

Tuesday marked the 3 week post-surgery, halfway point in recovery for this stage of my treatment. And it has been rough. I knew that going into it, but I never thought that losing my hair would be easier than surgery. I have just been so limited in movement that I am about to go crazy! I cannot move my arms to do even the simplest of tasks like emptying the dishwasher or getting a shirt off a hanger; I have been sleeping (stiffly and on my back only – no moving around!) under a blanket on the wrong side of the bed, since I cannot reach the lamp on my side with my right arm; and I have only recently been cleared to shower, so yes I stink a little. I could've handled all that with no problems, except one......I cannot pick up Charlie, feed him, change his diaper, or play with him like I used to. And it kills me.

I have to admit to a little depression coming from being around him and NOT being able to take care of him like I want to. The whole "This hurts me more than it hurts you" expression that parents use on their kids is ringing some-what true for me now. The saddest sight to see is his sweet little arms reaching up for me as he butt-scoots his way over to where I am sitting and I have to tell this one year-old that Mommy can't pick him up right now. It frustrates the hell out of both of us.

I've been trying not to let it get to me (too much!) and be as positive as I can under the circumstances, since I know it is only temporary and he won't really remember "Cancer Mommy" at all. I play with him as much as my arms will let me and I have graduated to feeding him his snacks since I can put pieces of banana or cheese on his tray without making a big mess. I have even tried taking my mind of my limitations by doing un-Charlie related things – I have some un-posted blog entries with my thoughts about the "New Jersey Housewives" show and the difficulties of only wearing buttoned-own shirts.......yeah, those will probably REMAIN unposted.

But today, the halfway point in the recovery period, I found pinwheels and everything changed.

Charlie is obsessed with pinwheels; he calls them "roun roun" for "around and around", which of course is what they do. My neighbor across the street has a pretty flowerbed in front of her house with about 7 of them and Charlie loves looking at them. He will point to them constantly and the closer we get to one, the more excited he gets. And when the wind kicks up......well, let's just say I may be getting a preview of what he will look like when he gets his first baseball bat/hockey stick/guitar/bicycle, 'cause this kid just freaks out! All the ladies in my family have been on a mission to find them to put in our yard and have managed to find only one in our search. UNTIL NOW.

Since I had also been cleared to drive, I decided to go buy some girlie essentials (mascara and shampoo YAY, Fantasy Football magazines....hey, I've got 2 drafts on Sunday and I need to read!....and other unmentionables). I figured asking Jesse to get them could result in wrong brands and possible embarrassment in the check-out line, plus I could get comfortable behind the wheel again on the short trip to Walgreens and back. While I was there, I looked in their seasonal aisle for pinwheels, hoping that they could have some left over in their discounted summer items before all the school supplies took over. Nope. So, I bought my supplies, checked out, and got in the car to make my way home. Then I passed a Family Dollar on Gallatin Road and figured they might be just the place to stock them. I entered, found the summer seasonal aisle with coolers, floats, water guns and ....JACKPOT! They had a ton – fabric ones that look like flowers, small plastic rainbow colored ones, and shiny tulip and butterfly shaped ones. And they were 40% off.... at the Dollar store. Finally the search is over! I bought as many as I my cancer arms could carry and went home as giddy as a school girl. Charlie was napping, so Jesse's mom and I planted them in the yard and were wild with anticipation for him to wake up and see the pinwheel wonderland we created for him. It was like Christmas morning.

While we waited for him to wake up, I realized that I felt

like I was his mom again. His proper mom. I may not be able to feed him or change him, but I know what he likes and I want him to know it. Cancer can prohibit me right now from hugging him, but it did a lousy job of keeping me from loving him in other ways. As we took him outside and I saw his smiling face at the sight of all the "roun rouns", I decided to not be funked out by my limitations and use what I got right now to the best of my abilities. What I got is a brain, a heart, and a whole lotta love for this kid. And now I got a lot of pinwheels.

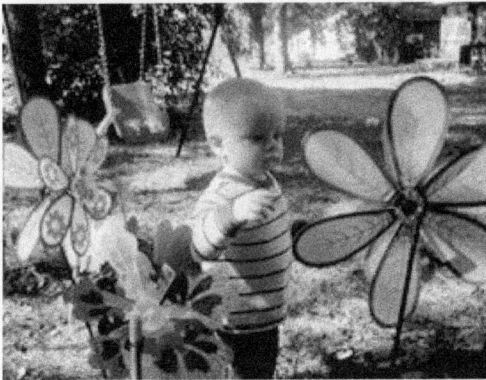

Charlie Loves the Roun-Rouns

It's Positively Cancer
August 28, 2012
Status Update for Week #4 Post-Surgery:
Last week I met with my oncologist for the first time since my surgery and there was good and okay news. The good news is that they are pretty sure they got all the cancer cells

out – the tumor and the 18 (!) lymphnodes that they saw are gone. Radiation should take care of the microscopic cells left behind, if there are any. She was confident that my surgeon was thorough in her search and that it hasn't spread anywhere else.

The okay news is that I still run a high risk of reoccurrence, given my Stage III status and the fact that there were more cancerous cells than previously believed. She has recommended that I participate in a clinical trial for another cancer-fighting drug called Erubilin, which has shown to stop the growth of cancer cells, but has only been FDA approved for cancer that has spread and not localized cancer like mine. This drug may not kill it for good, but it puts another bullet in the gun and will hopefully drop my reoccurrence percentage from 35% to something much lower – the goal here is under 20%. So, in a nutshell……I am starting 18 weeks of more CHEMO tomorrow. The side effects are about the same as the first go-around, but I got a lot of "maybes" on it: "maybe" I'll be nauseous, "maybe" I'll lose my hair again….great…., "maybe" my energy level will be low. The only certainty is that it'll be a lot more doctor visits and it will go on for the remainder of the year. So, during my 6 weeks of radiation which will be 5 days a week, I'll also have chemo once a week (even though I skip every third week) since they have told me that I can have both this kind of chemo and radiation at the same time. Wheeeeewwwwww……I'm exhausted just thinking about it.

It will be a long and busy week, as I get started with all this. I had out-patient surgery yesterday to put my chemo port back in (they took it out during my mastectomy), chemo tomorrow, and I go in for radiation-prep on Friday so they can mark me for the laser. By my birthday on Saturday, I will be a nauseated, no-boobs, unshowered port-scarred lady with Sharpie Xs all over my chest......how hot is that? But, on the bright side, my 35th year will be over and 36 will be the age that I beat cancer. That is my oncologist's plan and I'm on board. Good-bye 35 – Hello 36!

It's Positively Cancer... shared a link.
September 5, 2012
Way to go Kellie Pickler! Bringing awareness to us young ladies with breast cancer AND looking hot doing it! Bald is Beautiful! (it kinda makes me miss my sleek look......well, kinda.)

Now this is friendship. Kellie Pickler appeared in a video clip on Good Morning America Wednesday sporting a very different look: a totally shaved head.

The country starlet buzzed off her blonde locks on Tuesday in support of her best friend, Summer Holt Miller, 36, who was diagnosed with breast cancer in June and is starting chemotherapy treatments on Thursday.

"Cancer does not discriminate," Pickler said in a release. Added Miller, "If this compels even one person to change their mentality toward waiting until the age of 40 for their mammogram, then it will be worth it."

Miller — who has a family history of breast cancer — has always been vigilant about self-exams, and asked her doctor for a mammogram when she felt something might be wrong. After doctors did find a tumor, the mother of two underwent a double mastectomy, and was declared cancer-free in August (her chemotherapy treatments will help ensure the cancer doesn't come back).

It's Positively Cancer

September 7, 2012

Newly updated status….. here's the deal:

No more chemo. It has been a rough 10 days, for sure. I can go into the gory details and emotional highs and lows, but here it is in a nutshell – my stage of cancer doesn't qualify me for the trial to get extra chemo. Apparently I am in a weird middle ground: I have too little cancer to get the FDA approved drug which is for VERY advanced cancer, but I've got too much cancer to get the clinical trial version of it. Soooooo….I'm charging ahead with the treatment plan we started with, 30 days of radiation and 5 year drug therapy (non-chemo, pill form). The sucky part is I got my port put back in…..for no reason. Luckily, my surgeon and oncologist have been very apologetic and have waived most of the cost this put on us (probably due in part to Jesse calling them out and being quite upset by this change in plans – he is my consument cheerleader and he has a smart businessman brain, so he knew how to eloquently tell them how much this puts us out – emotionally and slightly financially – without it getting too dramatic).

It would only be natural to celebrate the fact that I have no more chemo, but I feel a bit of a loss with this development. I guess I thought that it was an extra security blanket for any kind of recurrence. I mean, Voldemort has to be slain for good, right? I have to admit to being confused, frustrated, dejected, and I am slightly questioning the fact that I can live through this, for real. My oncologist has said that my 41st birthday is going to be very huge, because that is when the high-risk window for reoccurrence starts closing. I have never in my life looked forward to being 41! It is no death sentence, but you never know how it works out.

But.....things are looking promising, so fear not! My plastic surgeon says everything is healing nicely and even injected some saline into my expanders to pump me up. I am still lumpy, but have some boobs now! Plus I got cleared to pick up Charlie and go about being "normal" YAY!! Radiation is on track and all things are "go"!

What I want to do now is live every day to the best of its ability. In light of all this, Jesse and I have decided together that we are doing something enjoyable every day; we figure that if we start now, it'll be natural after a few months and besides, who doesn't want to do something that is fun every day for the rest of their lives? If anything positive comes out of cancer, it is that we are living fuller lives. So, 2 days ago we started: Charlie stayed with his Gramma Hamilton overnight, so we saw a movie in the theatre for the first time since

Charlie was born. Yesterday, I cheated and rocked Charlie to sleep for his nap when I wasn't cleared for it (if only Victor Cruz would have had some kind of Fantasy Football blowout, the day would've been amazing!). Then today Jesse and I treated ourselves to lunch in Midtown and saw Barry Trotz (the Predators Head Coach)!

Life is so good when you live it in the present......

Give this 5 minutes to remind you what you should....... SEIZE THE DAY!!! Carpe Diem!

It's Positively Cancer
September 16, 2012
Look out Mia Farrow ...... I'm coming after your look!

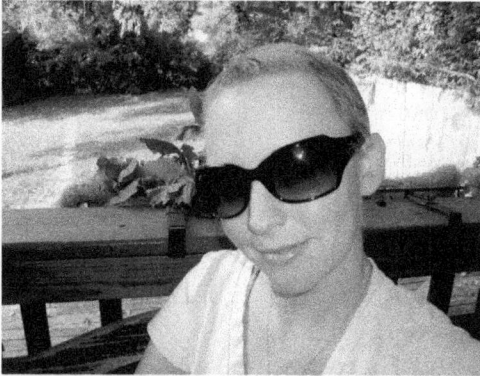

It's Positively Cancer
September 26, 2012
Okay fellas, I'm starting this post with a slight disclaimer for you. I am going to talk about boobs and bras, but it is not going to be very sexy. I just wanted to let you know up front

just in case you want to keep your romantic image of breasts intact. Okay? Good. If you keep reading, awesome, but don't say I didn't let you know ahead of time.

Being that I have breast cancer, the topic of boobs is a common one for me. I find it funny that I have become comfortable not only talking about my own breasts, but also comfortable with everyone fleetingly (or not so fleetingly, in some cases) glancing at them when in conversation with me (I can only guess that they are checking out my plastic surgeon's handiwork and luckily he has done a great job so far!). I have to take my shirt off so much around doctors and nurses who are perfect strangers to me that I have completely gotten over being shy about it. In fact, I may be becoming a bit too casual about it; I think I have embarrassed some people on more than one occasion by giving them waaaayyyy more information than they bargained for. Oops.

That being said, here is some info on how my breast reconstruction is going to work. During my surgery, my plastic surgeon had put in temporary expanders in place of my breasts to gradually stretch my skin to prepare me for the more permanent implants. Each time I see him, he fills them with saline a little at a time until we eventually get to the size we want. Then, after my body gets used to the stretching and is completely healed from the surgery, the implants go in. Sexy, right? This process takes about 6 months......and yes, for those dying to know, I get to choose the size I want to be.

So at my last appointment, I was inquiring about getting new bras for my new boobs. I am not allowed to wear underwire bras while the expanders are in, so I needed to know where I could find bras that fit my situation and could hold these heavy things in place. He told me of a boutique in the hospital called "Pretty in Pink" that is specifically designed for breast cancer patients going through treatment. Perfect! He wrote out a "prescription" describing my stage of treatment and the fact that I had a double mastectomy, and I was on my way to buy new bras for a new me.

The boutique itself is very small and completely hidden by foggy-glassed double doors that opened up to a hospital waiting room it was connected to. As I walk in, I am surrounded by pretty lacy bras, pink-ribboned emblazed T-shirts and bumper stickers, and frilly lingerie items. Not too bad! Two ladies are there to help me and since I had made an appointment ahead of time, we got started right away. They take me to the back dressing room area and closed not one, but 2 curtains to shield me from view from the shop. Very discrete, unlike what I have been used to so far. Without hesitation, I took off my shirt to get ready to be fitted. I realized that I was kind of excited about this shopping excursion – not only will I get something comfortable for these heavy expanders, but, as any girl will attest to, buying a pretty bra is fun and makes us feel, well, pretty! I stood there, anxiously waiting as the girls measure me and go to the back of the store to search their boxes for the right size. Then they found some, Eureka! From around the corner of the curtained dressing room, they ask me if I would like white or black. How about one of each? Yay, fun! They finally come back in to the small dressing room.......holding the biggest old lady bra I have ever seen. WHAT?! Come ON! What happened to all those lacy ones I saw hanging in the shop? I mean, these straps are Velcro, for crying out loud! How on earth am I supposed to wear a v-neck shirt or any kind of feminine top with THAT big thing underneath?! To make matters worse, they inform me that it is supposed to be a little loose in the cup size, since I am not at my full "potential" yet. To my horror, it dawned on me that I wasn't buying just a bra......I was getting a Training Bra. Oh. My. God. I am 13 years old all over again. I felt like I needed to get out an old copy of "Are you there God? It's me Margaret" and remember the days of braces, crushes on boys, and waiting for my period. How embarrassing.

I slip this monstrosity on and allowed the girls to fuss over the fit, completely disheartened that my fun girlie shopping trip was, well, not as much fun as I thought anymore. Bummer. But, the bra turned out to be very comfortable and it held the expanders in nicely without the heavy feeling they had been giving me. As I turned to look at myself in the mirror and saw my cancer boobs being held up by this cancer bra, all I could do was sigh and let it go. If cancer has taught me anything at all, it is to expect the unexpected, no matter how great or how small, and adapt to whatever comes my way. I have tried to learn to accept that things don't always turn out the way I think they will. I guess I am still learning that lesson.

The helpful ladies assured me that once I got the implants

in, I could come back for the lacy bras in the front of the store. I smiled at them, got dressed, and met them back out in front of the shop. Surrounded by racks of pretty garments (of which, I noticed, did NOT hold any of the bras I was holding......back of the store, indeed!), I paid for my new comfort bras, one in black and 2 in white. Jesse was waiting for me and asked how everything went. I gave him a smile and said "Great!". And I realized that I meant it.

I mean, after all, he's a guy – what does he know about training bras anyway?

It's Positively Cancer
October 10, 2012

Since it is Breast Cancer Awareness Month (I'm sure most of you are "aware" of this if you shop at Kroger and have seen all the pink products or are a football fan watching big burly men wearing pink socks), I feel a need to mention it here and make it known what I am doing for it. There are many things that anyone can do; buy said pink products at the grocery store, wear a pink ribbon in solidarity, and even donate time or money to the breast cancer charity of choice.

I have decided to do a few things ….. and it's not wearing pink all month, so don't look for a wardrobe change. Instead, I have signed up to be a volunteer at the American Cancer Society's "Making Strides Against Breast Cancer" walk that is taking place on Saturday October 20th at LP Field. They haven't quite told me where I will be exactly yet – I told them that I have experience in the food industry and can work a food booth, but I have a feeling from the vibe I am getting that I will be placed in the survivors tent. That's cool too, since apparently you get to meet other women living with breast cancer, from the newly diagnosed to the survivors in remission, and we can all meet, talk, and support each other. Talking is also in my comfort zone, so it sounds like a great way to pay it forward.

Then I started thinking.....I am happy to do this, but most of the people coming to the walk have already been affected by breast cancer. If we need to spread awareness, shouldn't we target those unaffected in order to make sure that ALL women are aware that they can be affected by it too? Especially younger women, who are not getting mammograms or think that they are too young to get cancer and don't routinely check themselves in the shower. Younger women are more apt to having a higher stage of cancer simply because they don't think that it can happen to them (hellooooo – I am Stage 3 at the age of 36, for crying out loud!).

So here's what I am doing – on Wednesday October 24th, my bar The Village Pub & Beer Garden is throwing a "More Birthdays!" party and we are going to donate 50% of our sales for the day to the American Cancer Society. I figure that a good portion of our clientele who come in drinking are, on average, between the ages of 21 – 45. That is the age group that is considered young for getting cancer. Why not provide possible life-changing/saving information in an environment that they are comfortable in?

If anyone reading this would like to come, everyone is invited. Please pass this along to anyone you feel would like to give their support. All you will be doing is drinking beer, giving to charity, spreading awareness, and hanging out with me. Can you think of a better way to spend an evening?

It's Positively Cancer
October 15, 2012

It's official – I now have a hairdo. I worked at the Pub over the weekend and had not one, not two, but THREE people talk about my hair without knowing that it was a chemo grow-out.

One of these encounters went something like this: I was walking by a table on the patio doing my manager thing (making sure everyone had full beers, empty tables were cleaned, the music was at a good volume, etc.) and the lady sitting there glanced at me. She apparently took note of my short hair and said to her companion something along the lines of "That's what I need to do, cut my hair short like that!" Her hair was dark brown and shoulder length and I guess their conversation prior to me walking up was about change (I am probably wildly speculating here, but this is my story so I'm going with it). I told her to go for it and we ended up talking about the perks of having short hair – low maintenance, quick drying, and, since she is a mom too, easy to deal with when you have small children. She even asked me who cuts my hair and I honestly told her my salon's name that I usually go to before cancer showed up, even though I was careful to word my answer to where I wouldn't state that it was the salon that cut it for me.

As we talked, part of me wanted to tell her the reason why my hair was so short. But why? Maybe I am so used to talking about cancer that it seemed natural. Maybe I wanted to give her the honest answer. Or maybe I have been validating the shortness for so long that I felt the need to explain that as a cancer patient, THIS is what you deal with. But then I realized something…..she had no idea I was a cancer patient at all. She just liked my "hairdo" and thought I cut it in a short pixie on purpose. To me, that means that I don't have to explain anymore about cancer merely because of my appearance. I can speak of it more voluntarily or NOT AT ALL if I choose. It is very freeing to know that now I have a choice.

Ahhhhhhh………..The light at the end of this cancer tunnel is shining more brightly every day……and my hairdo looks good in the sunlight!

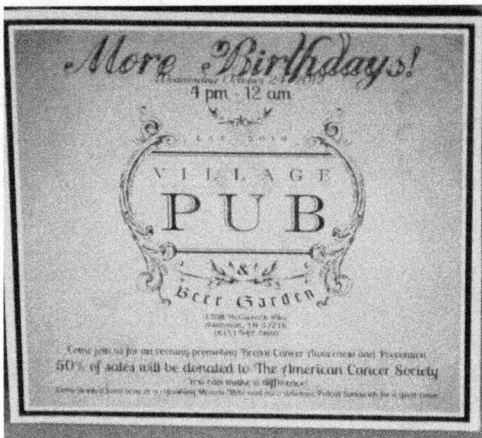

It's Positively Cancer shared Village Pub & Beer Garden's photo.

October 24, 2012

The Pub's Breast Cancer Benefit is tonight! I am so excited to be able to give back and hopefully help spread awareness to young people. If you guys want to come down for support (or just to have a beer and see how long my hair has grown !) the doors open at 4pm for Happy Hour 1/2 off drafts! Thanks for being supportive already by reading this blog – your comments have helped me get through the past year holding my head high and keeping my spirits up when I was low. Thank You!

Tonight's the night – our benefit for the American Cancer Society begins when we open the door at 4pm for Happy Hour! We will be donating 50% of our sales to the ACS's Making Strides for Breast Cancer program, so stop by for a beer and help us raise money for a great cause!

It's Positively Cancer

October 25, 2012

A big THANK YOU to everyone who came out to the Pub last night to raise money for the American Cancer Society! It warmed my heart to see so many friends, both new and old, come out to support breast cancer awareness and, in some sense, me. The final total everyone helped to raise is $1,643.64 – sweet! This will be one of the best checks I will write in a long time Thanks again everybody!

It's Positively Cancer

October 30, 2012

After 28 sessions, I am proud to announce that, as of today, I am officially done with radiation treatment!! I have realized that I had not written much about it and I was starting to wonder why. I can only explain that by saying that there was simply nothing to write about it because it was pretty boring. Nothing at all like chemo, which was somewhat social and gave me a chance to talk with the other patients or nurses. Radiation, however, is very isolated. I went in every morning at 10:30am, undressed from the waist up, laid down on a thin operating table under a big machine, and, after lining me up properly with all the markings I have on my chest, the nurses leave the room to work their radiation magic. It takes about 10 to 15 minutes, or the duration of about 5 songs that play on the radio in the room, and it doesn't hurt. I then get up, say thank you, get dressed and go on about my day. This was every day Monday through Friday for about 6 weeks. Granted, however boring it was, it became a bit of a chore after a couple of weeks. But the nurses were very pleasant and I got to see a chemo buddy every once in a while, so all in all, aside from the sunburn I'm rocking on my chest right now, it wasn't that bad.

When I first began this treatment, I decided to take a good look at my diet and see if I could do anything on my own to help the radiation really take effect. I felt that missing out on extra chemo was a bit of a let down, so I figured maybe there is something I can do during radiation that could give me the extra "bullet in the gun" that I was expecting from more chemo. I got a few books about eating properly when fighting cancer and basically took from them the information I knew I could use in my daily life. Most of the advice was common sense and I was pleased to find out that I did a lot of it already. "Eat your veggies, especially the green leafy ones" was one and since I have been a vegetarian for 15+ years, I had that one covered. "Salmon is wonderful for a good protein source with fatty oils that are great for you" is another and I have been gobbling it up like a crazy woman (I allowed seafood into my diet when I turned 30). "Shop the outside perimeter of the supermarket and you will avoid the processed foods from the middle aisles" – smart and good to know. I've also been taking probiotics to digest everything better, drinking Green Tea to help my immune system and water to keep hydrated, eating garlic in everything, and I even cut back on butter, opting for more olive oil alternatives since olive oil is crazy good for you. I figure, if I am going in every day to radiate my body, why not help it out, right?

All of it has been great and pretty easy, except for one thing – sugar. During my research into this cancer-fighting diet, I uncovered the fact that cancer cells LOVE sugar. It is like fertilizing a plant – it helps them to grow and flourish by giving them what they like to feed on the most. Okay, I thought, I'll give that up completely. I've never been a big dessert person anyway and if this can help my treatment work more efficiently and potentially help me beat cancer, then I am on board, no questions asked. So, no more candy coffee in the mornings, no more stealing a few Oreos from Jesse's supply that I buy him, no more sweet breads, ice cream, or even gum if I could help it. I even gave up my beloved Sprite, of which I am an addict of. If I am going to do it, I'm doing it all the way! I thought it would be a bit time consuming but not too hard – just read the label on everything and if there is any sugar in it, you can always find a 0 sugar alternative. I have never seen so many labels in my fridge with the words "sugar-free" or "no sugar added" in my life. I have even found LIGHT BROWN SUGAR for baking, ….. WHAT?! I threw out anything sweet in our kitchen that would tempt me and created a pretty good sweet-free area. Take that, cancer!

Then a couple of weeks into it……the sugar cravings hit. Oh My GOD, did they ever. Suddenly, every sugary, chocolaty, decadent dessert looked AMAZING. Commercials advertising cinnamon rolls or milkshakes or Reese's Peanut Butter Cups made me want to lick my television screen. We would talk about the wonderful gourmet ice cream sandwiches from (you guessed it!) Sugar Wagon that we sell at the Pub and it was all I could do to keep myself from getting one out of the freezer and gorging myself on it. And (save me now!) the holidays are approaching, so there are more temptations just waiting around the corner. Sigh.

Through all of these intense cravings, I have found sugar solace in one thing, yogurt. I spoke with a dietitian in my radiation office about sugar and she said that if there are benefits in some foods that out-weigh the sugar drawbacks, don't worry about it so much. Yogurt's live active cultures are so beneficial; I have cut myself some slack and I buy the low-fat kind. And I go all out....the have the BEST flavors of yogurt right now! Strawberry Shortcake! Pineapple Upside-Down Cake! Boston Cream Pie! Key Lime Pie! It is HEAVEN!!!!! Charlie is a big fan of yogurt too and he always looks up at me when I am eating it, expecting me to share with him. However, I have been Mean Mommy and horded it all to myself, even going so far as ignoring his urgent groans and obvious reaches towards my yogurt container as I shovel it in right in front of him. It is all I have right now, …. sorry kid.

But now that radiation is over, I can give myself a break. I won't go back to sugar-filled coffee drinks every morning, but I will allow myself a piece (or eight) of candy on Halloween or a slice of pumpkin pie on Thanksgiving for sure. I feel that the radiation has now done its job and the cancer cells should be, according to plan, dead dead DEAD, so there is nothing left for sugar to feed. So what is a bit of sweet, chocolaty goodness every once in a while going to hurt? (Seriously, agree with me on this one….. I'm twitching with urges no person should ever have that doesn't include another person) I have suffered enough this year because of cancer and deserve to indulge myself on occasion now that treatment is over (right?). And not only this treatment, but ALL the major treatments are done. YAY!!! That in itself is something to celebrate.

And I think I hear a piece of Malt Cake from Dalt's calling my name……..

It's Positively Cancer
November 16, 2012

What do these appointment cards all have in common? THEY ARE ALL FOR NEXT YEAR!!!!!!!!

Wednesday marked the last doctor's appointment I will have until February 2013. I am in the "Wait and See" phase, meaning that now that all the treatments are done (aside from the implant procedure that will take place sometime in the spring, but that is purely cosmetic), I just take a pill a day and see each doctor every few months to make sure I am feeling alright. The longer this goes without any major complications, the better my chances of remission.

And boy am I glad not to go to a hospital every week for something – what a relief! It is the perfect time too; this holiday season I will be able to concentrate on normal Christmas stuff rather than work around cancer like I have been doing all year so far. I think Santa has already brought my present to me! YAY!!!!!!!

It's Positively Cancer
November 21, 2012

It's a day early, but here's what I am thankful for after this crazy year:

Eyelashes

Pinwheels

Morning messy hair

Doing a push-up (I did one…..or 10!…..girl ones, on an incline standing up, but stilll!)

Gene Wider in "Willy Wonka and the Chocolate Factory" (Charlie LOVES this movie and I appreciate his brilliant performance keeping me interested every time I watch it, which is now once a day)

My Family, My Family, My Family

A wonderful best friend

A new family member on the way

Pubs and Beer!

It's Positively Cancer
December 17, 2012

Sorry I haven't been posting lately: I've been enjoying a much needed break from thinking/talking/being "cancer patient" that I have not felt the urge to write anything cancer related as of late. To be honest, I have been way too busy with getting back to a regular life to have any cancer stories to share anyway. Charlie is getting bigger and talking….a lot (Lord help me, he is such a parrot now, YIKES! This Mommy has to REALLY watch what she says now). Jesse and I took a wonderfully fancy "let's treat ourselves after this crazy year" vacation to the Biltmore in Asheville the week after Thanksgiving and spoiled ourselves rotten for 5 whole days – yes, there was expensive cognac, shotgun shooting at clay pigeons, a candlelight tour of the mansion, and ALOT of decadent food! And to top that off, we are buying a bigger house and starting another business. WHEW!!!! If I ever wanted to distract myself, I think I have found many outlets to forget that I ever had cancer to begin with. It has been really nice to live a regular life again. That IS the goal, right? After all the treatments, hospital visits, and schedule-juggling from meeting said appointments, the most blessed thing in life for me right now is just living a normal day-to-day life. However mundane it can be, I am beginning to love every bit of it. I get to spend time with my son and see him grow. I get to see my husband flourish in his career and truly be happy with his job and his role as a provider. I have the privilege of having all of Charlie's grandparents nearby so he can really get close to them and learn at a young age why I love them all so much – they are cool, loving, adventurous, and everything I will eventually be to him when he becomes an adult and realizes that I am not just "mean mommy". I have even taken a "behind the scenes" role in my career and have accepted that…. Charlie has a parent at home and that is the most important job I could ever have and am lucky enough to do (to any strong career-driven woman reading this, let me tell you this – KIDS.ARE.WORTH. IT! There is a reason why pro-athletes say "Hi Mom" or "I Love You Mom" …being a mom is the hardest job with the best pay-off – we get shout-outs on TV, the BEST hugs, and moms ALWAYS end up looking cooler than the dads do!) Yes, it was a much needed break. But the cancer cloud doesn't go away – at least not for 5 years, in my case. Doc says my 41st birthday is a big one and I am sure no woman has ever looked more forward to turning 41 than I am. I have had my youth and it was glorious.........bring on 41! Until then, I will take my daily "still kicking cancer's ass" pill, live out my life in the moment like Charlie does, and never EVER take life for granted. So, as one likes to look toward the future and wonder what the next year will bring, my holiday wish and New Year's Resolution for everybody (and mostly myself) is this: to live each day as it comes; to tell your loved ones that you love them every day; to do something fun every day to make each day fulfilling; and never, EVER take for granted the health that we are blessed with. Merry Christmas and I hope 2013 is a wonderful New Year for you all!

Do Something Fun Every Day!!

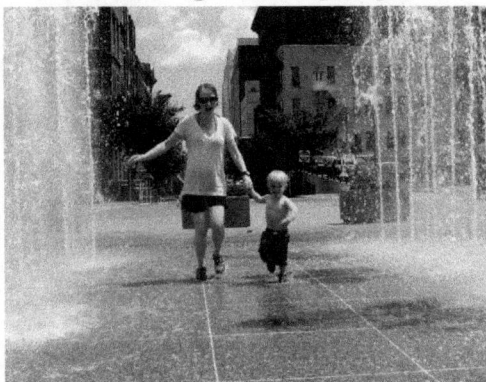

It's Positively Cancer
December 25, 2012

This Christmas, I am glad to reflect on the year as a challenging but learning year......I learned that your health really is everything, your family is the best friend you could ever wish for, and that life is the most amazing gift you have ever been given. And also that eating with your hands with gusto is the only way to truly enjoy food.

Merry Christmas to everyone who has supported me through cancer this year. God bless you and thank you from the bottom of my heart!

It's Positively Cancer

January 1, 2013 ·

Happy New Year! I know it is tradition to make resolutions right about now and I have always been one to, well, NOT do that. Why set myself up for disappointment when I don't meet these goals? Why give myself unrealistic levels of achievement? I know myself well enough to understand that I have probably set the bar too high with my past resolutions anyway and found it frustrating or inconvenient to "exercise 7 days a week" or "volunteer at a homeless shelter". So, long ago I decided to never make resolutions again and just be satisfied with living the next year out happily with out putting myself through the stress of not achieving the goals I set January 1st.

I have now changed my mind.

I was thinking about it all wrong. Why not challenge myself? Why not start off a new year with reasonable goals that could improve my quality of life and enhance my experience of it? And after this past year of full-on cancer craziness, why not give my mind something else un-cancer related to focus on?

The worst that could happen is that I could come out a better person for it.

So, with this in mind, here are Tracy Hamilton's first-in-a-long-time New Year's Resolutions for 2013:

Play

Eat

Walk

Give

Laugh

Write

Hug

Think kindly

Say yes

Pray

Be adventurous

And lastly.......love big and show it

I hope the new year brings wonderful experiences, lots of love, and good health to all of you too! (God I love the optimism of a fresh new year!!)

It's Positively Cancer
March 11, 2013

So I think I have mentioned that this is my year of giving back....especially to everyone I should have thanked (and hopefully did but never enough to my liking) for helping with Charlie care, support in general, and for being cool with a young cancer patient when she (me!) was in the throws of trying to figure all that cancer craziness out. I feel that the support I have been given over the past year could never amount to my gratitude and never-ending appreciation for the wonderful family I am not only privileged to be born in, but also blessed to marry into. So I am going to do it, one person at a time:

I showcased my wonderful dad and his book "My 7 Days In Heaven" (seriously people, buy this book, what a fun, thought provoking read!)

.....now check out my youngest sister Rosemary competing in a CrossFit Games competition. I watched this video amazed at the strength that this woman (and I KNOW HER!!!) has to completely physically and mentally rock this out! Truth be told, I am stunned that she can do this …. Not that I ever had doubt in her, but I just never realized how strong a woman's body could be and I have to admit, I am inspired! Rosemary has always marched to a cooler drummer and has never faltered from who she is, never compromises for what she believes in, and always been herself no matter what life throws at her. She is a positive thinker, influential motivator, and obviously one hell of a personal trainer! I told my Nashville-based trainer that I would love to have Evangeline Lily (circa 2003) "lost" era arms.......yea.....never mind. I want Rosemary circa 2013 arms now. Go Rosey Go!

It's Positively Cancer shared *Making Strides Against Breast Cancer- Nashville, TN*'s photo.
April 18, 2013
Here's proof that cancer has made THIS self-proclaimed

tomboy like pink and embrace feather boas...... AND, if anyone wants to come to this "Fabulous Females Fighting Cancer" fundraiser for the American Cancer Society on April 26th, BRING IT ON!!!! It should be lots of fun – there's wine, beer, food, a silent auction, and music from the WannaBeatles! You can buy your $30 ticket here – www.fabulousfemalesfightingcancer.org

It's Positively Cancer
May 20, 2013

It has been 6 months since I finished my treatments and boy have we been busy! We bought a new house, are starting a new business adventure, and we are working hard to keep up with the growing Pub business. Charlie is bigger and has been talking up a storm – as a mom, I can (and will!) brag about the fact that he is forming 4/5 word sentences and expressing opinions about things verbally too ("No like doggies", "Milk is good, tasty", and one of my personal favorites "Come on!"). My sister Kelly gave birth to a breathtaking, beautiful baby girl Drew Isabella, so I am once again an aunt! Yep, it has been a great time in our lives to build toward our future while enjoying the present.

But....... the honeymoon is over.

Last week I went to the doctor with a dull aching pain in my pelvic area that was shooting down my leg and generally causing a noticeable degree of discomfort. I went to my OB-GYN and after determining that I wasn't pregnant and that my cervix looked good, she said she felt something hard where the pain seemed to originate from. After an ultrasound and a CT scan, my doctors discovered 2 masses on my ovaries. I was sent to an OB-GYN Oncologist (another new doctor!) and after examining me and my ultrasound pictures, he determined that I need to have my ovaries and my uterus removed. As in, removed this Wednesday morning at 6:30am.

So here we go again. It is unclear whether the masses are breast cancer spreading or ovarian cancer until we get in there and look (I mean, are either one of those options better than the other? Geez!). It is going to be a full on hysterectomy and they will also be looking at the lymph nodes to make sure they get any infected ones out as well. I have also met with my breast cancer oncologist and she said we will form a plan a couple of weeks after the surgery once we know what we are dealing with. It is likely that more chemo will be involved, but exactly how much or for how long has yet to be determined.

I guess life has thrown me yet another curveball. I have to admit to some disappointment and lots of frustration about having to do this all…..over……again. I had a brief moment of "Why Me?!!!!!!" thoughts and feelings and I cried for myself a bit, but now I am just pissed off. And I mean Really. Pissed. Off. What the fuck, cancer, leave me alone! You've got my breasts and now you want my ovaries? Well, just slap a penis on me a turn me into a dude, why don't cha! My resolve to beat it once and for all has strengthened tenfold and I am determined to do whatever it takes to get rid of it for good. Luckily, my doctors are right there with me, hence the quickness of the surgery, and this go-around, we are going to work with their treatments along with complimentary natural, at-home remedies as well. Cancer is about to get its ass kicked (again), T-Rock style.

I will be recovering at the hospital for 3-5 days and then be at home for 6 weeks before we move on to the next stage. For now, Voldemort will have his day, but the magic is strong within me too. It's time to bust these Horcruxes once and for all.

It's Positively Cancer
June 2, 2013
Status Update:

It has been 1 week since I've been home from the hospital after my surgery and it has been alright, considering. I am not allowed to pick up Charlie for 6 weeks (big frustrated sigh) and I am a very slow mover. I had to stay in the hospital for about 5 days, which wouldn't have been so bad if they would've let me eat something (I mean, for real! This vegetarian would've gladly eaten a cheeseburger wrapped in bacon wrapped in steak wrapped in MORE bacon I was so hungry!). I was on a clear liquid diet FOREVER – it started the day before surgery when all I could do was drink water, tea, coffee, or some juices all day. After surgery, the doctors would only let me swab my mouth with a wet sponge on a toothpick......for 3 days. Seriously? They are concerned with your stomach and bowels, since they are shifting back into place and filling the void my removed ovaries and uterus left behind, and apparently your insides can be very sensitive during this process. Finally, I got to graduate to popsicles and a few sips of water here and there for a day and then, once they deemed that my body was situated enough to handle it, I got jello, vegetable broth, and coffee. Needless to say, I was glad to go home and slowly get back to eating, even if it is small portions of bland food for a while.

So, what was the outcome of this whole ordeal? I am happy to say that it was the best possible scenario! My surgeon said that it looked like it was the breast cancer that developed in my ovaries (NOT ovarian cancer, thank goodness!) and that it had not spread anywhere else. Being that my type of breast cancer is estrogen positive, I assume that it can sometimes go to the ovaries (I'll have to double check with my oncologist), but since it was NOT in any lymph nodes they were able to get it all. YAY – finally something positive, right?! I don't know what this means for any future treatments I may receive, but hopefully it won't be quite as intense as the first go around. I am seeing my oncologist Thursday morning to go over the results of the surgery and to see what our next plan of action is, so I will have more of an idea then.

It feels a bit odd to be celebrating the fact that breast cancer was once again the culprit for yet another lady part of my body being taken from me, especially one that now leaves me with no hope of ever having another child of my own. I mourn that, but I realize too that there was probably a slim chance of that ever happening anyway. Still, there was hope and now that is gone. But, if I start to feel sorry for myself and think that I am no longer a woman without boobs and a womb, I will remember what my wonderful husband said when I said that to him – "sure you are; you are a mother and a wife". What a keeper, huh?

Keep all fingers crossed that my oncologist will keep our plan of action more on the preventative side than the attack-and-kill methods from before (I cling to the thought that I MAY get to keep my hair!). Thank you to everyone who came to visit me at the hospital and for all the flowers that decorated my room, making the nurses love coming in to smell the "florist shop". You all rock and I love you for it.

Now, excuse me while I get down to fixing myself some brothy soup with a piece of plain white bread to eat.......because "as God as my witness, I will never be hungry again!"

It's Positively Cancer
June 10, 2013
Quote of the day: *"I didn't survive cancer, I defied it to try and take me!"*
(Thanks random comment guy on Facebook!)

It's Positively Cancer
June 10, 2013
New boobs! New boobs!!
We (meaning mostly my doctors, since I have been ready for this for months) have deemed it time to remove these

heavy, cumbersome expanders that I have been carrying around with me since August and finally give me my permanent breast implants. For those wondering what exactly expanders are, they are implant-type bags that are temporarily placed where your breast is to gradually stretch your skin to the desired size (and yes, I got to choose the size!). These bags are made of heavier material than an implant and are filled a little at a time with saline. Those who have a breast removed (like me) need these before implants because there was so much removed that your body and your skin need time to adjust – it's like getting braces tightened every few months in order to get straight teeth.

Well, I have cursed these damn things forever; they are truly uncomfortable and so weighty. They don't move at all and feel like bags of sand lying heavily on my chest, causing me to walk a little stooped over from the weight of them (at least, I feel like I do, my posture is awful!). I even have to sleep with my arm on a pillow if I sleep on my side because the gravitational pull on my arm pulls my body on top of them and adds more weight.....again, that is what it feels like to me. Plus, they are crooked and don't look the least bit natural. Not that it won't be somewhat obvious that I have fake boobs with the implants, but still.

So these suckers are coming out – tomorrow. Yep, another surgery for me, almost 3 weeks after my last one. This one isn't so bad, however. It is out-patient and they said most people resume normal daily activities in a matter of days not weeks. I won't be able to lift anything for 3 weeks, but I couldn't lift Charlie for about that long from my hysterectomy anyway, so that works out well. And the best part.....I will have a better quality of life and the weight of another surgery looming will be lifted off my chest, literally. It is the best kind of surgery this girl could ask for.

My oncologist decided to get this done now in order to plan for the next phase of my battle. As it turns out, even though they "got it all out" during the hysterectomy, she is afraid that the cancer may be an underlying one that could pop up quickly, unexpectantly, and randomly. She wants to monitor me closely to catch anything that is abnormal super early. That includes a couple of PET scans over the next few months to see if the cancer is anywhere else and possibly taking part of clinical trials. More chemo may not be the right move for me (it apparently didn't work perfectly to begin with), but we will see. I am doing my part too – I am eating my cancer-fighting foods, drinking kombacha and green teas, and taking turkey tail mushroom supplements every day. I will start exercising regularly as soon as they let me (I am ashamed to admit that I was lazy about that) and this bar owner even gave up alcohol (Good-bye beer! I will miss you!). Whatever I gotta do to get rid of this once and for all, I am on board.

First things first – new boobs! I can't wait to not have to wear a bra and maybe even have some cleavage! Jesse can finally have some of his wife back too........wink wink. Wish me luck and ladies, there may be a "Showing Off The New

Girls" party being planned for the end of summer – keep your calendars clear!

It's Positively Cancer
June 22, 2013

I have been marked as a Princess. This is a true story (bear with me here if I go a bit too long):

Back in my early twenties, I worked as a cocktail waitress at the Boundr'y restaurant for a few years and became great friends with a bartender named Jimbo. The Boundr'y, in those days, had a wild, but sophisticated bar scene known for its big martini pours, pretty clientele, and flirtatious atmosphere. The bartenders were all male at the time and extremely good at their jobs; not only did they make sure guests were well attended to with drink and conversation, but everyone was also made to feel rich, pretty, and above all, special every time they came in – especially the ladies. And Jimbo was one of the best. He was famous for his wild stories, his off-color jokes, his penchant for anything weird or adventurous, and his crazy haircut (a dyed blond mess of hair on top with the rest of his head shaved and a small Asian tattoo smack on the back of his scalp that meant "Mom"). Not really what you may imagine as a lady-killer type, but boy did his schtick work for him – the girls just love a bad boy.

One night we were working together and it wasn't too busy, so I was observing the master at work. The bar was shaped as a half-circle and he was at one end flirting with a group of ladies. As a cocktail waitress, I worked the tables around outside of the bar and as I passed by the group, I heard Jimbo call one of them "Princess" as he turned to go and make their drinks. The girls giggled and batted their eyelashes at his backside, eagerly awaiting his return. As I check on my tables and make my way to the other end of the bar, I spy Jimbo once again holding court with yet another gathering of pretty girls, all of whom had their glossy smiles and suggestive eyes firmly fixed on him as he flirted and poured. He made his drinks and turned to leave to deliver them, leaving these women with an "I'll be right back, Princess" line of some kind or another. They in turn swooned and giggled, nestling into their bar stools with their martinis until he came back. All I could do was roll my eyes – again with the "Princess"? Are girls THAT easy? Not all women wanted to be princesses when they were little (thank you very much!). But it obviously works for him and they love it.

At the end of the shift as we were closing up the bar, I make a few jokes about him using his special princess line on the ladies. He looks at me, shrugs his shoulders, and flatly told me that their names were not important enough for him to learn because they didn't mean anything to him but something pretty to look at or a big tip. Calling them "Princess" allowed him to flirt without any of the fuss that would require him to get to know them, even on a very basic level. "Princess" didn't mean special, as these ladies liked to think it did – it meant the complete opposite for Jimbo, un-special. Well, the surprise from his remarks must have been written all over my face (he was totally messing with them and they were completely clueless!), for when he looked at me, a sly grin spread all over his face and for the next few weeks, all he did was call me Princess. I was offended at first (dude, you KNOW my name and I am NOT falling for your little flirtatious game because I know better!), but after a while it became an inside joke between us.

A few months down the road, I decide it was time to get a tattoo. I wasn't sure exactly what I wanted, so I asked Jimbo for his thoughts. His eyes lit up like fireflies in summer and he excitedly suggested that I get "Princess" tattooed on me. He looked up the Asian characters for the word and pushed the idea on me for a few days. I have to admit, I liked the Asian version and, at the time, I was young enough to think an ironic tattoo is clever and fun. So, I agree to do it and Jimbo and I go see our tattoo artist buddy Timmy at his shop. 30 minutes later, the Japanese symbol for Princess is tattooed right below my belly button and Jimbo is as giddy as a school boy. "You will never forget me now!" I remember him exclaiming as we go out for celebratory new tattoo cocktails.

Fast forward to 6 weeks ago..........

I am sitting in my OB-GYN oncologist's office and he is explaining to me how my hysterectomy surgery will go. He informs me that he will be making an incision vertically from my belly button straight down until he reached my pelvic bone so he could basically open me up like a book and get a solid look of what he needs to remove. As I am digesting all of this information, he gives me a pitiful grin and lets me know that this incision will probably go right through my tattoo and he cannot guarantee that it will look as good as it did when they sew me back up. I told him that I understood, but I have to admit to being pretty bummed out by the thought – I have grown to really love this tattoo! It has become my memory of a good friend and a reminder of my wild younger days. But (sigh), I guess cancer has plans to spoil that for me too, damn it. Wellp, the surgery happens and during a follow-up exam at the hospital, my surgeon and his team of three are in my room to talk results and about how I need to take care of my incision, which was heavily bandaged and painful. My surgeon's assistant piped up that she took extra care in sewing me back up and seemed quite proud to relay that she thinks she did a good job lining up my tattoo. I gave her a weak smile and a thank you, but my expectations were not high.

I go home and after a few weeks the bandages start to fray and fall off. I am finally able to get a good look at my new scar. As I stand in front of the mirror to get the full effect, I was pleasantly surprised to see that the surgeon's assistant had reason to be proud – she did a wonderful job! Aside from the big red line going right through the middle, my tattoo looks almost as good as it used to. I turn from side to side admiring my seamstress's work and then it hits me – cancer didn't ruin this tattoo at all. It may no longer be exactly the Princess joke that Jimbo and I intended it as, but that is okay. My tattoo has a whole new meaning, thanks to you, cancer.

For now I am a Warrior Princess. And I have the permanent markings to prove it.

It's Positively Cancer

July 12, 2013

Whoo-Hoo, I've been cleared!! After 7 weeks (!) of surgeries and recovery time, all of my doctors have given me the go-ahead to resume a "normal" life (read: pick up Charlie again). My family has been amazing during this time helping to take care of Charlie and me, but I am crazy excited about my house ceasing to be Grand Central Station and getting some alone Mommy time with Charlie back again. I can now take him swimming, "play toys", and do errands without a chaperone – blessed freedom! Of course, since this is cancer that I am dealing with here, this freedom is still with its limits. While I can care for Charlie now on my own, I am still undergoing treatment. I had a brain MRI and a PET scan about 2 weeks ago so my oncologist could see if the cancer was anywhere else and we discovered that there was cancer in some lymph nodes in my back, which had been causing me lower back pain, and a couple of legions on my liver. The back pain was due to the lymph nodes swelling from the cancer and putting pressure on my kidneys, so we put in a (painful!) stint in the artery that goes from my left kidney to my bladder to keep the waste system of my body functioning properly. Now I have to temporarily deal with bladder infection type symptoms (awful, awful stuff!) and chew on Tylenol all day. But we have to keep the system flowing properly because......yes folks, wait for it......I have started chemo again. Yup, my first dose was last Friday and

I will get another in a couple of weeks. We are starting with just 2 doses to see if it works and shrinks the cancer down. If it does, great! If not, we will form another plan of attack. My oncologist doesn't want to waste time or money on a treatment that isn't working and I love that attitude! But, being that it is chemo, even 1 dose means I will more than likely lose my hair again and I will probably be bald by this time next week. So, in the spirit of turning chemo lemons into sweet, delicious cancer-fighting lemonade, Jesse and I had a date night with my hair on Tuesday. We got all gussied up – him in a fancy tie and dress pants, me in a dress I haven't been able to fit in since I was 25 (which was a weird dichotomy of a YAY moment and an I-am-way-too-cancer-skinny-for-this realization) – and we got driven around town in a big fancy black car from Grand Avenue Car Service. Dinner at the new "we are booked solid on a Tuesday night" Nashville restaurant Husk, which was one of the best dining experiences I have ever had. (Nashvillians, go there. Now.) Next we were on to Rock Bottom's roof top bar at twilight for a beer where we gazed over the bustling downtown Broadway action while simultaneously staring hypnotically at the high river lapping the shores of LP field. A visit to Pub 5 on 4th for a little re-con, Tootsie's for whiskey and, apparently, covers of classic rock tunes (where was the country music, people, c'mon!), and finally back home to East Nashville for our night cap. To truly sum things up, my hair lived it up and had a great night on the town – it got styled for dinner, tousled in the wind, smoked out in a bar, and frizzy in the summer evening air. Not a bad send off. The next day, while nursing a slight whiskey headache, I took good look at this recurrence, with all its surgeries, more chemo, and future hair loss and I surprised myself about how I've felt toward it. Sure I am still trying to push forward with a positive attitude, but I am less scared, more confident, and I truly believe it in my bones that this time, I am doing everything I can to win. Even if I don't. They say that when you are diagnosed with cancer that most people change, some for the better, some not so much. Most survivors develop an "every day is amazing and precious" type attitude. I have to admit to wanting that feeling when I was diagnosed, but I didn't totally buy into it until now. Maybe now I've made peace with cancer, maybe now I have learned to relax and live, maybe now I have gotten closer to God and let go of my worries. I believe it is all the above. So I don't fret about my hair loss, or chemo, or the fact that cancer is still here in my life. My lesson to learn is to pick up Charlie every day, do something fun every day, and be kind to people every day. To me, that is a life well worth living. Here is a "History of My Hair" from the past 2 years. See…..it grows back!

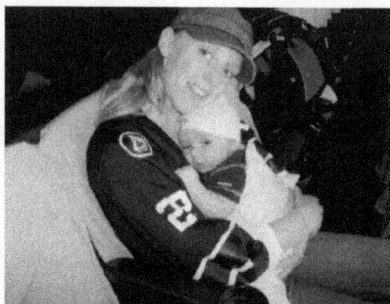

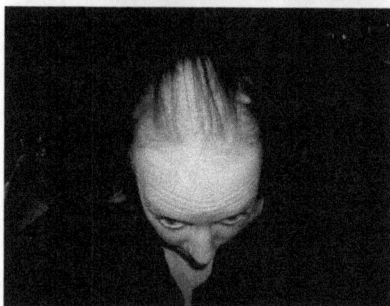

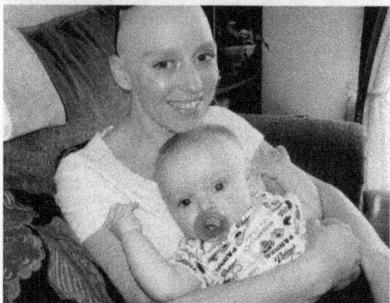

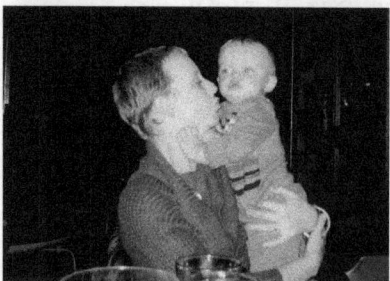

It's Positively Cancer

July 25, 2013

Check out who else is bald? I don't care what your politics are, this is a cool gesture (does this make my bald head more presidential? I choose to think so........)

This is AWESOME!! President George H. W. Bush joined members of his Secret Service detail in shaving his head to show solidarity for Patrick, who is the son of one of the agents. Patrick is undergoing treatment for leukemia and is losing his hair as a result.

It's Positively Cancer

July 31, 2013

I know I have named this blog "It's Positively Cancer", but I need to whine a bit. I have to admit to feeling a bit bummed out lately. This current stint with chemo is kinda wiping me out – I don't know if it is a harder drug or that this time I have 2 major and 2 minor surgeries under my belt, most of them recently. In fact, today marks the year anniversary of my double mastectomy, the first of them all. But, whether it is from the surgeries or not, I am tired and achy and I can't seem to get past it. I have leg pain that causes me to slowly move with a bit of a limp, backaches (since that is where cancer has decided to setup shop for now), my fingers are going a bit numb (chemo side effect), and I am getting a double-whammy of hot flashes, since both chemo and the hysterectomy causes them. Oh yeah, which by the way, I am 36 and going through menopause. Great.

Plus, I am catching glimpses of my reflection in windows and randomly placed mirrors and I keep realizing that I am bald again. I know, I know…..I have seen this look on me before and it is really nothing new. BUT, I thought that I was done with it and I had such a solid head of hair that took me a year to grow out. And to top it off, I am super skinny from all my surgeries (weighing in at a paltry 114 pounds…..and I have GAINED some weight!), so feel like I look cancery. I have been trying to gain my weight back, but since I am not eating sugar, every thing is low-fat and so good for me that it is a slow process. It is hard to imagine that in April, I was a healthy 126 pounds and had curls on the back of my head……3 months later I am a stick figure with a shiny dome of a noggin. I guess I am still in shock.

I think this time feels worse because now I know that there is a possibility that I could not only rock this look for a long while, but I may have to do it again and again. And no matter how nicely shaped my head is, I prefer hair, thank you! So, yeah, I'm feeling kinda bummed out. I didn't realize how hard I was taking this until the other night, as I was sitting next to Jesse on the couch, I got a hot flash and had to take my hat off to cool down. I turned to Jesse and asked pitifully "Do you mind if I take my hat off?" Yes I did. In the privacy of my own home, to my understanding husband who likes my head, I actually asked permission to fly the bald flag. Jesse looked at me with an exasperated expression on his face and gently said 'of course not". Then he paused as I sheepishly took off my hat and then said something like, "I wish you would have the same positive attitude you had the last time about your hair. You handled it so well." What a slap in the face. He was right (yes ladies, husbands can be right every once in a while). I was only making myself miserable dwelling on it and why do I want to do that? That is no way to live.

So, I am once again embracing my look. The aches and pains may still wear on me, but being depressed about my cancery appearance doesn't have to. So I decided to contact my photographer friend Lauren and we did a photo shoot at my house showing off my baldness and my skinniness. I felt like I should capture this moment in time in order to realize that this is part of my journey in life, and it is okay. With cancer, change is inevitable and I have come to realize that I will never be the same; in looks, in attitude, and in my outlook on life. Why not give it a big hug and accept it as not a bad thing, but something to learn from and grow on.

Huh.......I guess my whining was only temporary. I named my blog correctly after all!!

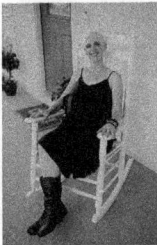

It's Positively Cancer
September 12, 2013

THANK YOU SO MUCH

It has been a rough 5-6 weeks and I certainly appreciate all the cards, flowers, birthday wishes and especially the letters detailing what is going on in your lives (keep those coming!). Due to complications from this recent cancer issue, my eyesight is temporarily not that great, so Jesse has been reading all these cards and letters to me every night before I go to bed – what a simple treat! I'm doing better, walking around pretty well and taking each day one day at a time. Truthfully, aside from my slow mobility and the fact that I can't see my hand in front of my face, I feel pretty great!

I thought I should post a quick "cancer hasn't knocked me down yet" update, so you all know I'm still alive and kicking! I really appreciate all the well wishes and hopefully I will be making my way back into the real world again soon. Here's a recent picture of me and all my pretty things that I can't see... I'm keeping my fingers crossed that the picture is good enough for Facebook.

Thanks Dad for typing this post out for me

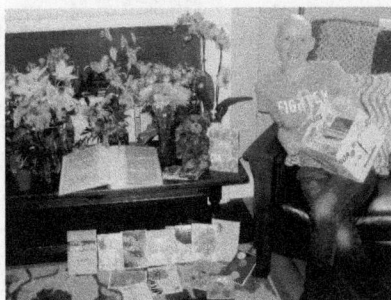

It's Positively Cancer

December 10, 2013

Dear Loving Friends and Family,

I'd like to post on behalf of the most wonderful friend and soulmate anyone could ask for, my wife Tracy. I was always so impressed with this blog and how well she expressed herself through it. This was very important to her as a conduit during her battle. It's just one of the many wonderful things about her that I've been blessed to be a part.

Today, she moves to a peaceful rest stop on the way to her final destination. As I write, she'll move to hospice and spend her final days in comfort surrounded by her loved ones. It's not the end we envisioned when this journey began, but the reality is that this will happen to us all one day. May we handle it with the dignity and conviction that's been her example.

Her battle was painfully fought at times, but always with strength and courage. At the same time, she was open and honest about her fears. The time for her to be afraid will soon pass, and for that I will be grateful. I will always miss her kind soul and her irreplaceable friendship. It feels like half of me is leaving, but if I follow her example, I know I'll see her again.

I love you so much, Hon.

Jesse Hamilton

It's Positively Cancer
December 16, 2013
Hello All,

I'm flattered and comforted by all the pictures, posts, and comments remembering Tracy. She truly was a wonderful, beautiful person, and the world will always be a better place because she was here.

Please read the obituary below, and make plans to join us to honor & celebrate at the service and the wake.

Jesse Hamilton

Obituary for Mrs. Tracy Lynn Hamilton

Tracy Lynn Hamilton, age 37 of Nashville, TN departed this life December 15, 2013 following a courageous battle with breast cancer. Tracy was born September 1, 1976 in San Diego, CA to Andrew Damien Smith and Debbie Paramore Raftery. She moved to her hometown of Nashville in 1983.

Tracy, above all, loved being a wife and mother. She enjoyed gardening and cooking and was an avid Nashville Predators fan. She loved football as well, especially fantasy football. She organized the Riverside Blossom Festival for two years and also helped organize *Fabulous Females Fighting Cancer.* She opened and operated three successful small businesses: Hamilton Bartending Services, Village Pub & Beer Garden, and The Hop Stop.

She is survived by her husband, Jesse; son, Charlie; parents, Andy Smith, Nancy Smith, and Debbie Raftery; sisters, Kelly Smith (Ben) Modena and Rosemary Barrow; niece, Drew Modena; and father and mother-in-law, Tom and Jennifer Hamilton; brother and sister-in-law, Andrew and Erin Webb and nephew, Henry Webb.

A celebration of Tracy's life will be conducted at 2 P.M., Saturday, December 21, 2013 from the Chapel of Spring Hill Funeral Home.

Interment will follow in Spring Hill Cemetery.

The family will receive friends from 10 AM until 1 PM on Saturday at Spring Hill Funeral Home.

A wake to celebrate Tracy's life will be held at 6 P.M., Sunday, December 22, 2013 at the Village Pub & Beer Garden, 1308 McGavock Pike, Nashville, TN 37216.

In lieu of flowers, memorial contributions may be made to the American Cancer Society

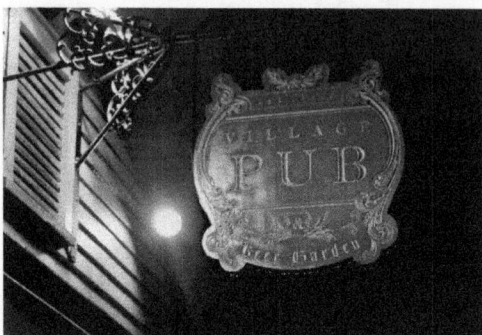

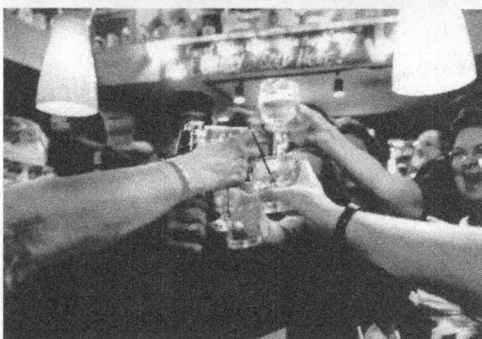

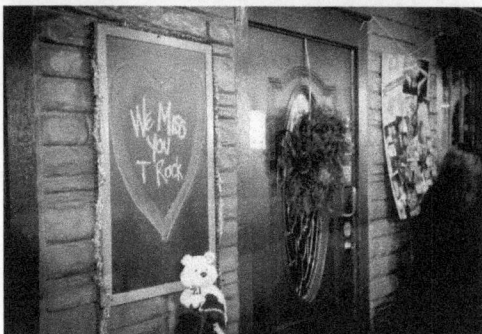

Wake – December 22, 2013 – Village Pub & Beer Garden

6

Dear Charlie

Dear Charlie;

It was the beginning of the toughest day of my life. The phone rang about 7am and I knew without looking what it was.

"Andy," said an emotional Jesse on the other end "I think it's time … you need to come"

It was December 15th 2013. I didn't sleep much that night and in fact, when Jesse called I had already been up and showered and ready to go. The night before when I left Alive Hospice, I knew that it wouldn't be much longer and I wanted to be ready for the call whenever it came.

When I opened the door to Tracy's room, I found Jesse quietly at her side holding her hand. He got up and we had a good hug. A quiet hug. I took my place on the other side of her and held her other hand.

Jesse briefed me on how the night went. Not much to report, really. Her breathing had become shallow with no

122 • Andy Smith

gasps or signs of discomfort. Mostly we just stood at her side and watched her. It wasn't more than a minute or two before Jesse softly spoke the words we didn't want to hear.

"I think she's gone."

I watched her chest... there was no rising... still... no expression ... no indication of life from this beautiful young woman that was my daughter and best friend for the past 37 years.

Jesse was right.... her suffering was over.

After a few very quiet minutes, I let go of Tracy's hand, kissed her forehead and went to the other side and simply held your Dad. All I could say was, "I'm so sorry Jesse"

Jesse called in a nurse who confirmed that Tracy had left us. She told us that she would hold off calling the funeral home to come get her until we were comfortable and left us to be alone with her again.

I asked Jesse if we should start calling family, but he looked at me with moist eyes of brokenness and said, "Not yet ... let's just sit here with her."

We sat there quietly for at least a half hour or so. I don't recall any conversations. Whatever was said was short comments of gratitude for having known such a woman. I think we both understood that we were the lucky ones. We got to experience the remarkable life your Mother lived. We got to see her at her best and at her worst and we both understood that even on her worst day you wouldn't want to be with anyone else. Even in her death, she was considerate enough to hold on until I got to her side. She was not going to leave your Dad alone. She needed her Dad to be with your Dad.

After a period of just being in the moment, Jesse decided that it was time to make the calls out to family. The phone call I never wanted to make.

Since most everyone was staying at Aunt Kelly's, I called her phone. I have no idea how the conversation went, but I know it was short. I didn't want to talk to Kelly, I wanted to hold her. Then I called my brother Mike as agreed so he could call the rest of my family. There was no way I wanted to make several calls in that moment.

Jesse and I went back to our quiet vigil of being with Tracy while we waited on family members to arrive.

The rest of the day is a blur. Lots of family …. lots of hugs … lots of decisions to follow schedules properly. All done with a heart so heavily burdened with sadness that simply breathing was exhausting.

I was so thankful your Dad took his time earlier to be still, be quiet, be alone with Tracy. Moments like this in life can quickly become busy with appointments, schedules and obligations to protocol. So many emotions creating such a variety of responses and actions that calls you into the depths of your compassion to accommodate everyone as best you can when all you really want to do is go away and cry.

A father should never be in a position to watch his daughter take her last breath, but if this is what I must bare, I will forever be grateful that I did so with your Dad. I can't imagine the heartache he endured on this day. I only know mine and it is beyond any words.

I lost a daughter that day.

Your Dad lost a wife he loved so very much.

Without understanding, you lost a mother you never had a chance to know.

That will always be the ultimate weight of sadness in my heart.

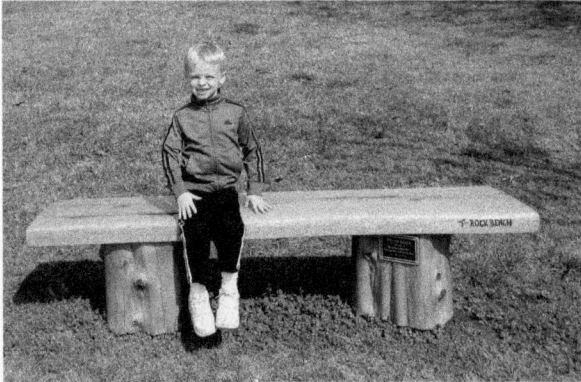

Charlie visits T-Rock bench Shelby Park, Nashville, TN 2017

The End

Thanks Tracy
for being so special

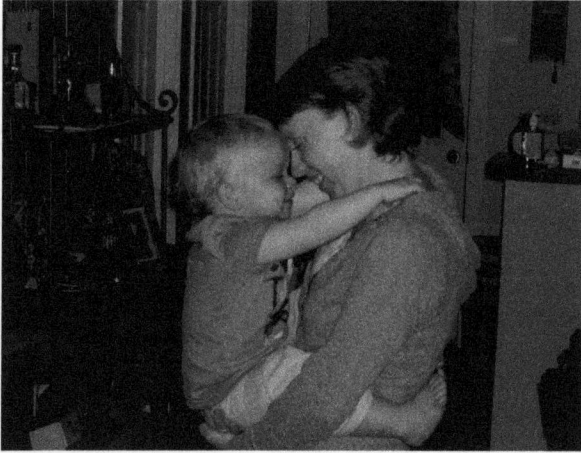

we will always miss you

www.ingramcontent.com/pod-product-compliance
Lightning Source LLC
Chambersburg PA
CBHW021833020426
42334CB00014B/610

* 9 7 8 0 6 9 2 9 9 2 9 6 8 *